The Pictorial Atlas of Common Genito-Urinary Medicine

Shiv Shanker Pareek
MBBS, Dip VD, Dip FPC, DTM&H
Associate Specialist in Genito-Urinary Medicine
London Road Community Hospital
Derby, UK

Foreword by
Professor Rob Miller

Radcliffe Publishing
London • New York

Radcliffe Publishing Ltd
33–41 Dallington Street
London
EC1V 0BB
United Kingdom

www.radcliffepublishing.com

British Library Cataloguing in Publication Data

A catalogue record for this book is available from the British Library.

ISBN-13: 978 184619 475 7

The paper used for the text pages of this book is FSC® certified. FSC® (The Forest Stewardship Council®) is an international network to promote responsible management of the world's forests.

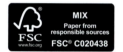

Typeset by Phoenix Photosetting, Chatham, Kent
Printed and bound by Hobbs the Printers, Totton, Hants

New research and clinical experience can result in changes in treatment and drug therapy. Readers of this book should therefore check the most recent product information on any drug they may prescribe to ensure they are complying with the manufacturer's recommendations concerning dosage, the method and duration of administration, and contraindications.

Contents

Foreword

'Life is short, science is long: opportunity is elusive, experiment is dangerous, judgment is difficult.'
Hippocrates of Kos, *Aphorisms*, Section I, i

'One picture is worth ten thousand words.'
Fred R Barnard, *Printers Ink*, 10 March 1927

Sexually transmitted infections (STIs) continue to be a major global health concern and are often associated with significant medical and psychological morbidity. The World Health Organization reports that over 340 million new cases of bacterial and protozoal STIs occur every year, worldwide. Additionally, UNAIDS estimates that globally, 33.3 million persons were living with HIV infection in 2009. In the United Kingdom the Health Protection Agency reported that in 2010, 418 598 new STI diagnoses were made in England; despite a slight reduction in total numbers of new STIs there was an 8% increase in diagnoses of syphilis and genital herpes and a 3% increase in gonorrhoea. In the UK in 2011, an estimated 86 500 persons are currently living with HIV infection.

Given this enormous global health burden it is essential that as well as genito-urinary and dermatology clinicians, others in primary care and casualty/emergency room settings, especially those in training or service-delivery grades, are able to recognise, diagnose and institute (or appropriately refer on for) timely treatment of STIs.

A book such as *The Pictorial Atlas of Common Genito-Urinary Medicine* which provides a comprehensive pictorial library of common and less common STIs, and which does not set out to replace or compete with the major textbooks of STIs, will facilitate these clinical activities. It will be of immense practical 'in the clinic, on the desk' day-to-day use for clinicians working in diverse primary and secondary healthcare settings anywhere in the world. Additionally, this picture atlas will provide a useful visual resource for both undergraduate and postgraduate students who are preparing for their professional exams.

Professor Rob Miller
London
October 2011

Preface

In the United Kingdom and Saudi Arabia, I have been practising, teaching and researching for more than 30 years in the field of sexually transmitted infections and conditions affecting the genitalia, which in modern terminology is known as genito-urinary medicine. During this time, I have seen patients affected with almost all types of diseases described in the standard textbooks on this specialty and I have never missed an opportunity to take a photograph of the cases that I have seen. Thus, over the years, I have accumulated a photographic encyclopaedia of genito-urinary diseases, which I have always thought would be an invaluable learning aid for medical students and healthcare professionals working in this field.

Genito-urinary medicine is a vast field that is associated with other specialties such as HIV medicine and dermatology. Since HIV, in a relatively short period of time, has become a separate discipline in its own right, I have focused my attention on the other aspects of the diseases within the genito-urinary field.

This book is not an attempt to supplant any existing textbook: its purpose is to provide a pictorial supplement to the standard works on the subject. It is an atlas of genito-urinary medicine, which embodies my lifetime hands-on experience in this fascinating field.

I thank the staff of the Department of Genito-Urinary Medicine and other staff at the Derby Hospitals' NHS Foundation Trust, particularly the Medical Illustration Department and my colleagues, Dr A Apoola and Dr R Rajakumar, for their advice during the writing of this book.

Last but in no way least, I must say that this book would not have been possible without the love and help of my closely-knit family, especially my wife, Meena.

Any feedback or comments on the content of this book would be greatly appreciated, either direct to me or via the publisher's website.

Shiv Shanker Pareek
October 2011

Acknowledgements

I would also like to thank Dr Pravin J Patel for providing ultrasound results, Dr Ranjeet Chaudhary and Mr Mike Cust for helpful advice, and Dr Scott Gouveia for editorial assistance during the preparation of this book. Various other sources of illustrations have been acknowledged in the associated captions.

I would further like to extend my thanks and acknowledgement to Dr Gwenda Hughes for allowing me to publish the SHHAPT Codes in this book which is in accordance with NHS Information Standard Notice (ISN) which is the official document.

I would like to thank Mr Paul Desmond, Executive Director of the Hepatitis B Foundation of UK: content was taken from the Green Book 2009.

Thanks to BASHH for providing permission to use extracts from the *International Journal of STD and AIDS* (GEG Group).

Thanks also to Mr REF Street for his valuable help in subediting the text and his work on the detailed preparation of the illustrations.

Dedication

This book is dedicated to my teacher and friend, Professor BR Madan, without whose inspiration I would not have written it.

Sources of information

The following sources, listed alphabetically, were used to check information and treatment guidelines:

- Bhutani LK, Khanna N. *Colour Atlas of Dermatology*. 5th ed. New Delhi: Mehta Publishing House; 2006.
- eMedicine website. Available at: http://emedicine.medscape.com (accessed 16 October 2011).
- Encyclopaedia Britannica online. Available at: www.britannica.com (accessed 16 October 2011).
- King A, Nicol C. *Venereal Diseases*. London: Cassell; 1964.
- Kingston M, French P, Goh B, *et al*. UK national guidelines on the management of syphilis 2008. *Int J STD AIDS*. 2008; **19**(11): 729–40.
- Lazaro N. BASHH CEG guidelines: which guidelines are popular? *Int J STD AIDS*. 2010; **21**(12): 847–8.
- MedicineNet website. Available at: www.medicinenet.com/script/main/hp.asp (accessed 16 October 2011).
- NHS Choices website. Available at: www.nhs.uk/Conditions/Pages/hub.aspx (accessed 16 October 2011).
- NHS Sexual Health and HIV Activity Property Type (SHHAPT). Available at: www.datadictionary.nhs.uk/data_dictionary/attributes/s/ses/sexual_health_and_hiv_activity_property_type_de.asp?shownav=0 (accessed 16 October 2011).
- Pattman R, Snow M, Handy P, *et al*. editors. *Oxford Handbook of Genitourinary Medicine, HIV and AIDS*. Oxford: Oxford University Press; 2005.
- Patel R, Alderson S, Geretti A, *et al*. European guideline for the management of genital herpes, 2010. *Int J STD AIDS*. 2011; **22**(1):1–10.
- PubMed Health website, available at: www.ncbi.nlm.nih.gov/pubmedhealth (accessed 26 April 2011).
- SHHAPT Code 2010 available at: www.isb.nhs.uk/documents/isb-0139/amd-99–2010/index_html, and the supporting material is available at: www.hpa.org.uk/gumcad (accessed 16 October 2011).
- www.hepb.org.uk (accessed 16 October 2011).

Chapter 1: Genitalia

1.1: Male internal and external genitalia (Fig. 1.1, next page)

1   **Urinary bladder** – collects urine prior to its excretion from the body. It has a capacity of approximately 500 mL. The daily volume of urine excreted depends on the level of hydration. The bladder comprises four layers: serous, muscular, submucous, and mucous. Inside the bladder, the trigone and internal orifices of the urethra and the two ureters are noticeable.

2   **Ureter** – each kidney has a ureter carrying urine from the kidney to the bladder. The ureters are each about 250 mm in length.

3   **Seminal vesicles** – these are paired glands located on the posteroinferior aspect of the urinary bladder. A major part of the fluid in semen is secreted by these glands. The secretion is alkaline in nature and contains fructose.

4   **Rugae** – these are multiple mucosal folds inside an empty bladder.

5   **Urethra** – this starts from the internal urethral orifice in the urinary bladder and runs to the external urethral opening at the glans penis. It is divided into three parts: the prostatic urethra, the membranous urethra, and the spongy urethra (also called the penile urethra). The total length of the male urethra is 175 mm to 200 mm. The urethra has two main functions: to allow urine to empty from the bladder and to allow the flow of semen during ejaculation.

6   **Prostatic urethra** – this is the part of the urethra passing through the prostate. It is about 24 mm in length.

7   **Membranous urethra** – this is a short section of the urethra between the prostatic urethra and the spongy urethra. The length of the membranous urethra is 10 mm to 15 mm.

8   **Spongy (penile) urethra** – this is the longest portion of the urethra, about 150 mm to 160 mm in length, and is located inside the corpus spongiosum penis. It runs along the ventral surface of the penis.

9   **Cowper's glands (also called bulbourethral glands)** – these are a pair of small glands situated posterior to, and lateral to, the membranous urethra. They secrete clear fluid which is added to semen.

10 **Epididymis** – this structure is present on the posterior side of each testis and is a coiled part of the spermatic duct which connects to the vas deferens. The epididymis accumulates and matures sperm cells and carries them to the vas deferens prior to ejaculation. The epididymis has three parts: head, body, and tail.

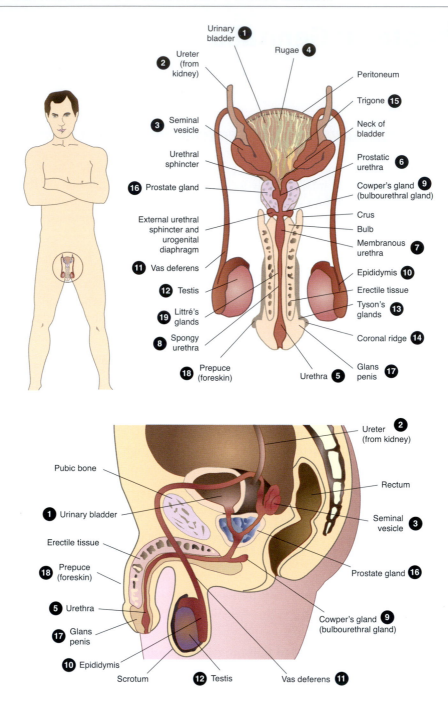

Figure 1.1: Male genital organs.

11 **Vas deferens** – this is a muscular tube which extends from the epididymis to the prostate, via the seminal vesicle, where it connects to the urethra. It carries mature sperm to the urethra for ejaculation.

12 **Testes** – there are two oval-shaped testes (singular: testis) within the scrotum. The spermatic cord starts from the top of each testis. The testes produce testosterone (the primary male sex hormone) and sperm cells. Testes contain seminiferous tubules in which spermatogenesis occurs.

13 **Tyson's glands (also called pearly penile papules)** – these are similar to sebaceous glands and are situated around the corona and inner surface of the prepuce of the penis. They are not always present and are not thought to be pathological. The glands may be analogous to preputial glands found in other mammals.

14 **Coronal ridge** – this separates the shaft of the penis from the glans.

15 **Trigone** – this is the internal triangular area of the urinary bladder between the two ureter orifices and the internal urethral opening.

16 **Prostate gland** – it contains two prostatic ducts which connect to the prostatic urethra. The gland produces fluid which is added to the ejaculate.

17 **Glans penis** – this is the head of the penis. It is reddish in colour, smooth and shiny. When the penis is erect, the glans becomes moist and very sensitive.

18 **Prepuce** – this is the outer retractable foreskin of the penis. Its function is to cover and protect the glans penis.

19 **Littré's glands (also called periurethral glands)** – these are situated in the urethra and secrete mucus which is mixed with semen during ejaculation.

1.2: Female internal and external genitalia (Fig. 1.2, next page)

1 **Vagina** – this is a muscular canal which extends from the cervix to the surface of the body. It is normally 150 mm to 180 mm in length and is lined by mucous membrane. The vagina has a few tiny secretory glands which lubricate it.

2 **Bartholin's glands** – these were documented in the literature in 1677. They are paired glands situated on either side of the lower ends of the labia minora near the vaginal opening. Each measures 10 mm to 30 mm in diameter and produces mucus via Bartholin's ducts when the woman is sexually aroused. An infected Bartholin's gland develops a Bartholin's abscess.

3 **Skene's glands** – these glands are also reported as paraurethral glands. They are present on the upper wall of the vagina near the urethra. They are close to the area described as 'the G-spot' and are analogous to the male prostate gland.

4 **Vestibule** – this is defined as the space between the labia minora and the opening of the vaginal orifice.

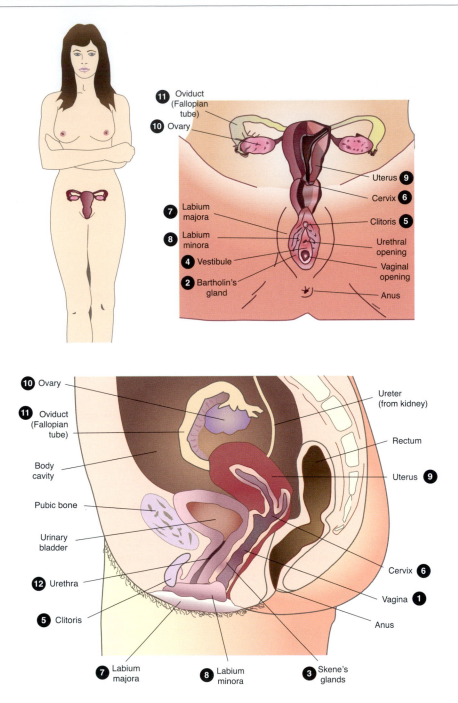

Figure 1.2: Female genital organs.

5   **Clitoris** – this is a very sensitive organ which is actually a bundle of nerves. It is the size of a pea and located at the top of the labia minora, 20 mm to 30 mm above the urethral opening.

6   **Cervix** – this is the narrow portion of the uterus which opens into the vagina. The segment of cervix opening in the vagina is called the external os. The segment between the external os and uterus is called the endocervical canal; this ends at the internal os.

7   **Labia majora** – these are two large folds which cover the labia minora. They are composed of fatty tissue and vary from woman to woman. They are often called the 'outer lips'.

8   **Labia minora** – these are a smaller pair of skin folds, often called the 'inner lips'. They vary from woman to woman.

9   **Uterus** – the uterus is a pear-shaped organ located in the lower abdomen between the bladder and rectum. The portion above the cervix is termed the corpus; it has two layers, a thin inner layer, the endometrium, and a thick, outer muscle layer, the myometrium.

10 **Ovary** – there are two ovaries, one on each side of the uterus, They produce eggs and female hormones. They are each about the size of an almond.

11 **Fallopian tube or oviduct** – each ovary is connected to the uterus by a fallopian tube (oviduct) which transports eggs from the ovary to the uterus.

12 **Urethra** – the female urethra is shorter than the male urethra and measures about 40 mm. It is situated above the front wall of the vagina and consists of three layers: an outer muscular layer, spongy erectile tissue, and an inner mucous membrane.

Chapter 2: Syphilis

History

Syphilis is a disease with a long history; it was present in the New World prior to 1492 and possibly introduced into Europe at about this time. There is some documented evidence of syphilis among sailors who returned to Europe from the New World in 1493, perhaps even by Columbus. Girolamo Fracastoro (1478–1553) is best known for giving the disease the name 'syphilis'; it was taken from an epic poem he wrote about the disease in 1530, entitled 'Syphilis sive morbus Gallicus', which translates as 'Syphilis or the French disease'. In 1905, Fritz Schaudinn (1871–1906) and colleague Erich Hoffmann discovered the bacterium that causes syphilis: *Treponema pallidum*. Prior to this, syphilis and gonorrhoea were thought to be caused by the same organism. The British physiologist and surgeon John Hunter (1728–93) reported that after he had inoculated himself with exudates from a patient with gonorrhoea, he developed gonorrhoea and syphilis. We now know that these diseases are caused by different bacteria and Mr Hunter's patient just happened to have both infections.

Causative organism

Syphilis is caused by a bacterium belonging to the *Spirochaetaceae* family. There are more than 70 species in the genera comprising this family, with some of the genus *Treponema* pathogenic to man, causing syphilis, yaws, bejel and pinta. Syphilis is caused by *Treponema pallidum* (Fig. 2.1), yaws is caused by *Treponema pallidum pertenue* (described by Castellani

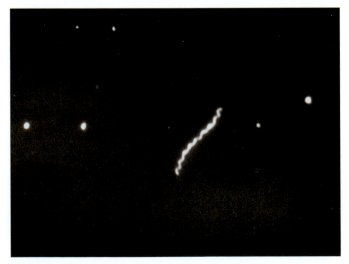

Figure 2.1: *Treponema pallidum.*

in 1905), *Treponema pallidum carateum* is responsible for pinta, while *Treponema pallidum endemicum* is the causative bacteria of bejel (non-venereal endemic syphilis).

Morphology

Treponema pallidum is a thin, spiral-shaped bacterium consisting of 8 to 24 coils. This organism is 6 μm to 15 μm in length and 0.24 μm in width, so is not visible with the naked eye. The motility of this organism is like the movement of a corkscrew.

Incubation period

Syphilis incubation period is 9 to 90 days.

Mode of transmission

Syphilis may be transmitted by:

- sexual contact.
- infected blood transfusion.
- mother to foetus.

Classification of syphilis

Syphilis presents either as a congenital infection (from birth, transmitted in utero from the mother), or as an infection acquired later in life.

Acquired syphilis

Acquired syphilis develops in four stages:

1   primary syphilis.
2   secondary syphilis.
3   latent syphilis.
4   tertiary syphilis (also referred to as late syphilis).

Primary syphilis

Primary syphilis typically presents as a painless syphilitic chancre or skin sore which may become ulcerated, and is contagious. Even if untreated, these usually heal in three to eight weeks. In addition to the primary chancre at the site of inoculation, primary syphilis is associated with regional lymphadenopathy (swollen lymph nodes).

Sites of primary chancre

- Extragenital sites
  - tongue.
  - nipple.

  – finger.

  – anus.

 • Genital sites – male.

  – glans penis.

  – shaft of the penis (Figs. 2.2, 2.3 and 2.4).

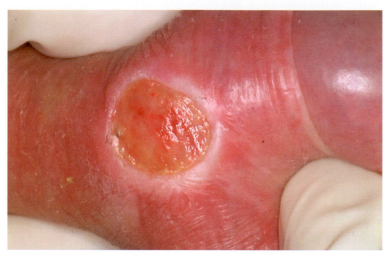

Figure 2.2: Primary syphilis: chancre.

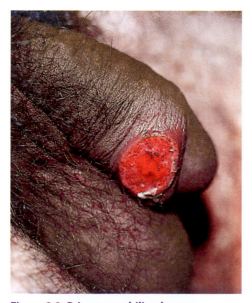

Figure 2.3: Primary syphilis: chancre. (Courtesy Dr N Khanna and Mehta Publishing House)

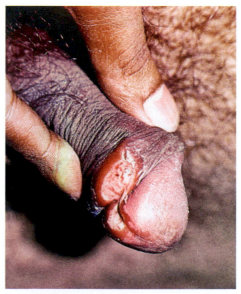

Figure 2.4: Primary syphilis: solitary indurated syphilitic chancre. (Courtesy Dr N Khanna and Mehta Publishing House)

    – scrotal area.

    – coronal sulcus.

    – perineal area (Figs. 2.5 and 2.6).

• Genital sites – female.

    – fourchette (Fig. 2.7).

    – between the genital and perineal area (Fig. 2.5).

    – cervical region (Fig. 2.8).

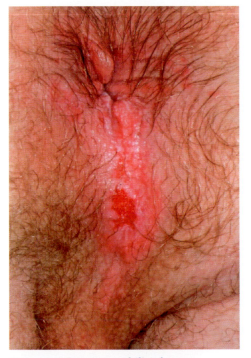

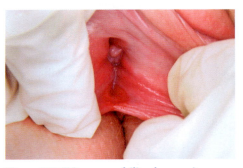

Figure 2.7: Primary syphilis: chancre in fourchette area.

Figure 2.5: Primary syphilis: chancre between the genital and perineal areas.

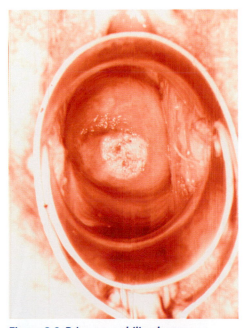

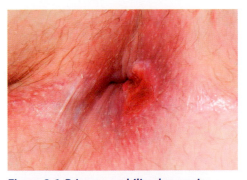

Figure 2.6: Primary syphilis: chancre in perineal area.

Figure 2.8: Primary syphilis: chancre on cervix.

- vulval area.
- vagina.

Diagnosis

- Dark-ground illumination of fluid from primary chancre to identify presence of *T. pallidum*.
- Aspirated fluid from one of the regional lymph nodes.
- Serological tests for syphilis (after four weeks from the appearance of the primary chancre).

Secondary syphilis

After the disappearance of the primary syphilis chancre, with or without treatment, symptoms of secondary syphilis will be evident within two years. The symptoms are:

- Skin rash.
  - generalised skin eruption (symmetrical) (Figs. 2.9 and 2.10).
  - macules, papules, nodules or pustules may be present.
  - palmoplantar syphilides (Fig. 2.11).
  - follicular rash.
  - papulosquamous rash.
  - nodular lesions (Fig. 2.12).
  - palmar syphilides (Fig. 2.13, page 12).

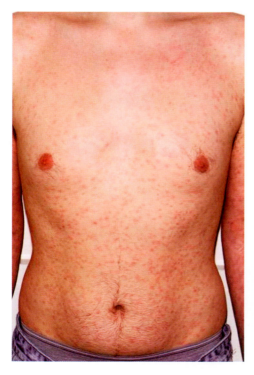

Figure 2.9: Secondary syphilis: rash on body area.

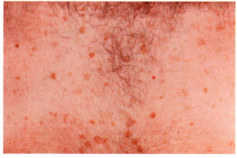

Figure 2.10: Syphilitic rash, in detail.

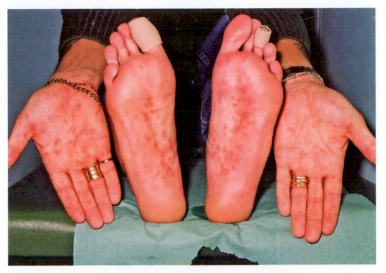

Figure 2.11: Secondary syphilis: palmoplantar syphilides.

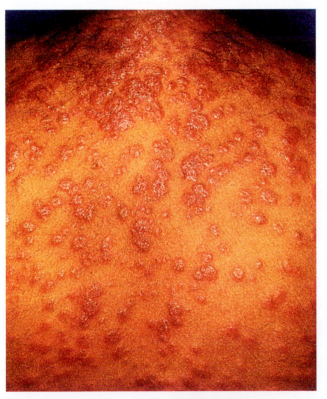

Figure 2.12: Secondary syphilis: nodular lesions, rare symmetrical pattern. (Courtesy Dr N Khanna and Mehta Publishing House)

- Pyrexia (low-grade fever).
- Lymphadenopathy (lymph nodes palpable).
- Liver involvement (abnormal liver enzymes and raised alkaline phosphatase).
- Mucous membrane ulcerative lesions (in the genital area) (Fig. 2.14) and snail track ulcer.

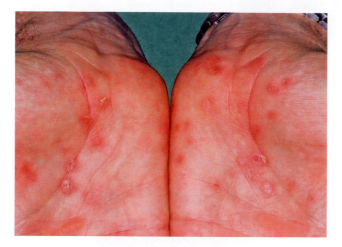

Figure 2.13: Secondary syphilis: palmar syphilides.

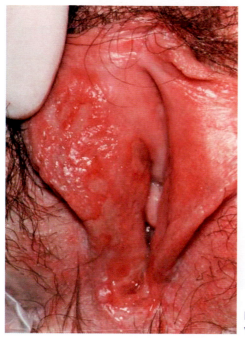

Figure 2.14: Secondary syphilis: ulceration in vulval area.

- Ophthalmitis (iridocyclitis – inflammation of the iris and ciliary body).
- Meningeal involvement (abnormality of cerebrospinal fluid).
- Oral lesions (erosive mucosal lesions) (Fig. 2.15).
- Alopecia, described as 'moth-eaten alopecia' (loss of hair) (Fig. 2.16).
- Condylomata lata (genital warts associated with *Treponema pallidum* infection) (Figs. 2.17 to 2.20, next page).
- Headache.
- Malaise.
- Periostitis (pain and aching in bones, muscles and joints).
- Neurological involvement (occasionally headaches and vomiting).
- Secondary syphilis: genital ulcers (Fig. 2.21, page 15), palmar syphilides (Fig. 2.22), and plantar syphilides (Fig. 2.23).

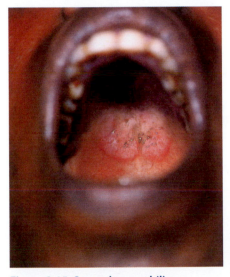

Figure 2.15: Secondary syphilis: erosive mucosal lesions. (Courtesy Dr N Khanna and Mehta Publishing House)

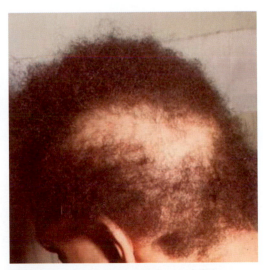

Figure 2.16: Secondary syphilis: syphilitic alopecia.

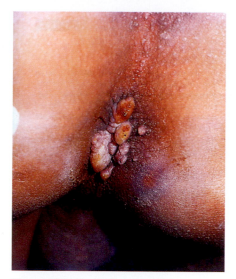

Figure 2.17: Secondary syphilis: condylomata lata perineal flat papules. (Courtesy Dr N Khanna and Mehta Publishing House)

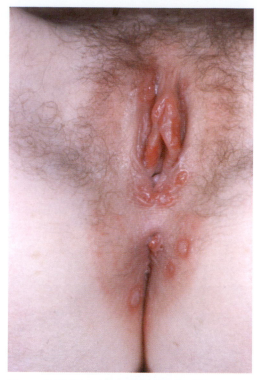

Figure 2.18: Secondary syphilis: condylomata lata. (Courtesy of CDC)

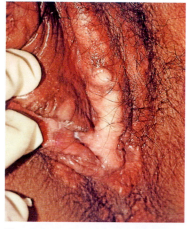

Figure 2.19: Secondary syphilis: condylomata lata perineal flat papules of vulva. (Courtesy Dr N Khanna and Mehta Publishing House)

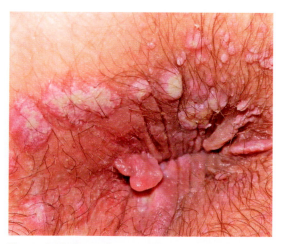

Figure 2.20: Secondary syphilis: condylomata lata papular lesions.

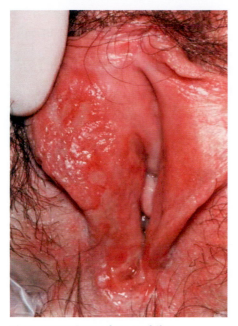

Figure 2.21: Secondary syphilis: genital ulcers.

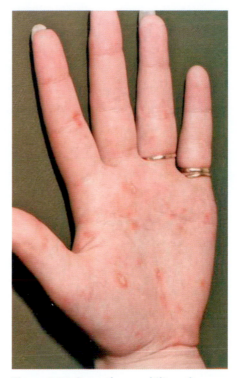

Figure 2.22: Secondary syphilis: palmar syphilides.

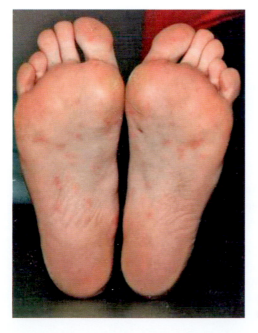

Figure 2.23: Secondary syphilis: plantar syphilides.

Diagnosis

- Dark-field illumination of fluid from ulcerative lesions or condylomata lata to identify presence of *T. pallidum* (Fig. 2.24).
- Occasionally abnormal cerebrospinal fluid (raised white cell count and protein).
- Liver function (including raised alkaline phosphatase).
- Reactive serology – positive results in serological tests including:
  - venereal disease research laboratory (VDRL) test.
  - rapid plasma reagin (RPR) test.
  - fluorescent treponemal antibody absorption (FTA-ABS) test.
  - immunoglobulin G (IgG) antibody test.
  - immunoglobulin M (IgM) antibody test.
  - enzyme immunoassay (EIA) test.

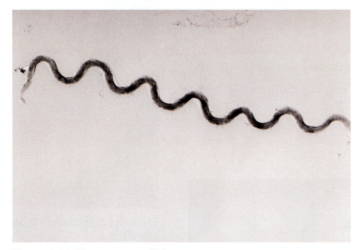

Figure 2.24: *Treponema pallidum.*

Latent syphilis

Early latent syphilis

This is the stage of the disease when the symptoms of secondary syphilis spontaneously recover (irrespective of treatment) in less than two years from the time of infection. There are no clinical signs or symptoms at this stage, but it is the most infectious stage of syphilis.

Late latent syphilis

If the symptoms of secondary syphilis spontaneously recover (irrespective of treatment) more than two years from the time of infection, the disease enters the late latent stage. Recurrence of symptoms is less likely during this stage than during the early latent stage.

Tertiary (late) syphilis

If untreated, syphilis enters a tertiary, or late stage in some patients, which may have cardiovascular and neurological elements. This stage is not infectious and usually develops three to ten years from the time of infection. Diagnosis of syphilis at this stage can be confirmed by serological tests, X-ray examination of bones and examination of cerebrospinal fluid.

Characteristic lesions are gummata – rubbery tumours – which may occur singly or in multiple, and do not contain *Treponema pallidum* bacteria. Gummatous lesions may be:

- nodular.
- squamous.
- subcutaneous.

Gummatous lesions usually occur on the tongue, skin, bones and mucous membranes (including the mouth), but may occur on any part of the body. Ulceration of oral gummata may lead to necrosis and perforation of the hard or soft palate (Fig. 2.25).

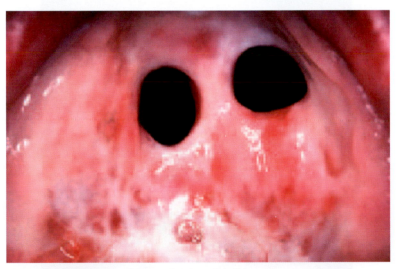

Figure 2.25: Tertiary syphilis: palatal perforations. (Courtesy Bains & Hosseini Ardehal)

Cardiovascular syphilis

Cardiovascular lesions may develop at any time from 10 years after the initial infection and may take the following forms:

- aortic aneurysm (marked degree of dilation of the proximal and distal aorta) (Figs. 2.26 and 2.27, next page).
- ruptured aortic aneurysm (Fig. 2.28, next page).

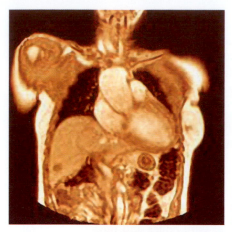

Figure 2.26: Tertiary syphilis: aneurysmal dilation of ascending aorta. (Courtesy of *International Journal of STD & AIDS*)

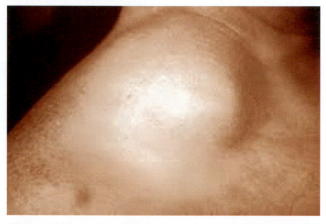

Figure 2.27: Tertiary syphilis: aortic aneurysm. (Courtesy of CDC)

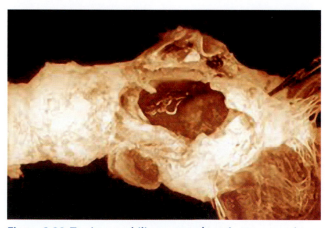

Figure 2.28: Tertiary syphilis: ruptured aortic aneurysm in cardiovascular syphilis. (Courtesy of CDC)

- aortitis – causing aortic regurgitation.
- Stokes–Adams' syndrome (gummatous lesions of the heart causing obstruction to the blood flow).

Neurosyphilis

Meningeal involvement may develop during the early stages of syphilis but it mainly develops in late syphilis. Although neurosyphilis may remain asymptomatic, many possible symptoms may be present, including:

- Argyll Robertson's pupil (small pupil in which the accommodation reaction to near and far objects is normal, but the pupil reflex to light is lost or reduced; previously referred to as 'prostitute pupil'. First described in 1869 by Douglas Argyll Robertson (Fig. 2.29).
- General paresis of the insane (paralytic dementia first described in association with syphilis by Esmarch and Jessen in 1857).
- Tabes dorsalis (Fig. 2.30) – degeneration of the myelin covering the nerves in the dorsal columns of the spinal cord, leading to the following symptoms:
  - Charcot's arthropathy – a neuropathic aspect of the disease causing degeneration of the joints; first reported by Jean-Martin Charcot in 1868

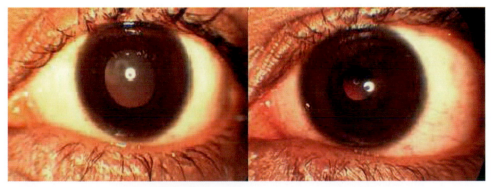

Figure 2.29: Neurosyphilis: Argyll Robertson's pupil. (Courtesy of Dr Nagpal)

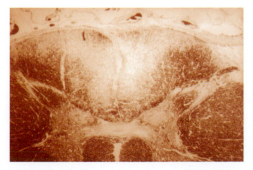

Figure 2.30: Tabes dorsalis. (Courtesy of CDC)

(Fig. 2.31, which also shows bismuth deposition – resulting from a treatment prior to the advent of penicillin).

– Ataxia (impaired balance and coordination) – Romberg's sign is positive (unable to stand upright with both feet together and eyes closed; first described by Moritz Heinrich Romberg in 1846).

– Dementia.

– Diminished reflexes.

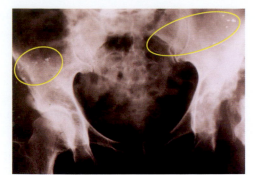

Figure 2.31: Neurosyphilis: Charcot's arthropathy affecting pelvic bone; bismuth deposition (highlighted in yellow).

Congenital syphilis

Mode of transmission

Congenital syphilis infection develops in the unborn foetus. The mother may have the disease and transmit it to the child in utero, or an infected father can transmit the disease to the child via the mother (as an intermediary). The syphilis bacterium passes through the placenta into the foetus causing congenital syphilis which develops in three stages:

1 early.

2 late.

3 stigmata.

After transfer of infection, the following adverse events may occur:

- miscarriage.
- premature birth.
- stillbirth.
- death of the baby soon after birth.

Early congenital syphilis

In early congenital syphilis, there are no primary stages (appearance of chancres) and no secondary stages (appearance of rash and ulcers in mucous membranes), and the infection can remain asymptomatic for up to two years (after which it is called late congenital syphilis).

- Symptoms of early congenital syphilis:
    - skin lesions – bullae (Fig. 2.32).
    - congenital syphilis skin lesions on the soles of the feet (Fig. 2.33).
    - syphilitic alopecia.

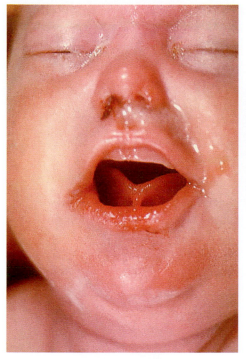

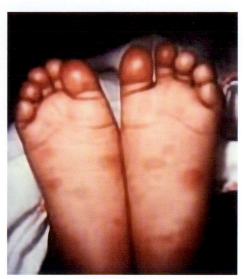

Figure 2.32: Congenital syphilis: skin lesions. (Courtesy of CDC)

Figure 2.33: Congenital syphilis: lesions on the soles of the feet. (Courtesy of CDC)

– lesions of mucous membranes.

– syphilitic rhinitis – or syphilitic 'snuffles'.

– nasal discharge.

– lymphadenitis.

– hepato/splenomegaly.

– neurological effects – stiffness of the neck, Kernig's sign.

– Bony lesions – osteochondritis.

– Ophthalmitis – choroiditis.

Late congenital syphilis

- Symptoms of late congenital syphilis:

– photophobia.

– iridocyclitis.

– neurological involvement, including juvenile general paralysis.

– meningitis.

– bony lesions.

○ sabre tibia – thickening of the middle third of the tibia.

     ○ Clutton's joints – symmetrical hydrarthrosis (accumulation of fluid) of the knees and elbows in congenital syphilis; first described in 1886 by Henry Hugh Clutton (1850–1909).

    – interstitial keratitis.

Stigmata

Stigmata of early congenital syphilis

Severe lesions from early congenital syphilis may leave long-term scarring called stigmata, which may cause deformity.

- Saddle nose (the bridge of the nose is absent).
- Hutchinson's teeth – deformed and notched incisors (Fig. 2.34) (in permanent teeth); first described in 1858 by Jonathan Hutchinson (1828–1913), and part of 'Hutchinson's triad'.

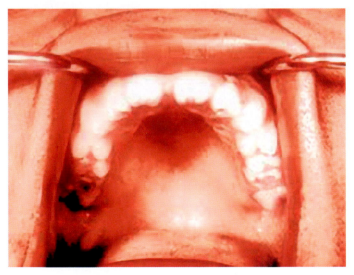

Figure 2.34: Hutchinson's teeth. (Courtesy of CDC)

- Hutchinson's triad:
  - interstitial keratitis.
  - Hutchinson's teeth.
  - 8th nerve deafness.

Stigmata of late congenital syphilis

- Interstitial keratitis.
- Gummatous scarring, frequently of the liver but also of the skin, heart, brain and bone.

- Optic atrophy.
- Periostitis of the sternoclavicular part of the clavicles, leading to Higouménakis's sign (thickening of the clavicle bones); first described in 1927 by George K Higouménakis (1895–1983).

Diagnosis of syphilis

Detection of organisms

Dark-field microscopic examination to show presence of *T. pallidum* bacteria in lesions.

Serological tests

Non-treponemal tests

These detect non-specific antibodies associated with syphilis infection.

- Venereal disease research laboratory test (VDRL).
- Rapid plasma reagin (RPR) test.
- Toluidine red unheated serum test (TRUST).

The following biological factors may lead to false positives:

- infectious mononucleosis.
- hepatitis.
- varicella-zoster (chickenpox/shingles virus).
- endocarditis.
- mycoplasma infection.
- pregnancy (in rare cases).
- cirrhosis of the liver.
- tuberculosis.
- autoimmune disease, including systemic lupus erythematosus (SLE).

Treponemal tests

These detect specific antibodies to *T. pallidum* and are used to confirm positive non-treponemal tests. Because of their specificity, a positive result may be obtained long after successful treatment for syphilis.

- Fluorescent treponemal antibody absorption (FTA-ABS) test.
- *Treponema pallidum* particle agglutination (TP-PA) assay.
- *Treponema pallidum* haemagglutination (TPHA) test.
- Enzyme immunoassay (EIA) test.

In rare cases, the following conditions may give false-positives to these high-specificity tests, but the less-sensitive non-treponemal tests should be negative:

- Lyme disease.
- yaws (a disease caused by a subspecies of the syphilis bacterium, *T. pallidum pertenue*).
- pinta (a disease caused by the bacterium *T. pallidum carateum*).
- leptospirosis (also called Weil's disease).
- rat-bite fever (caused by *Streptobacillus moniliformis* or *Spirillum minus* bacteria).
- pregnancy.

Diagnosis of neurosyphilis

The VDRL, TPHA and FTA-ABS tests are performed on cerebrospinal fluid (CSF) to diagnose neurosyphilis. CSF cell count, protein estimation and IgG index are also very important diagnostic tools. The RPR test is not indicated for neurosyphilis.

Recent developments in diagnostic tests for syphilis

- Immunoglobulin M (IgM) test – this test will confirm syphilis and congenital syphilis because IgM crosses the placenta. IgM antibodies may be detected by enzyme-linked immunosorbent assay (ELISA) or FTA-ABS test.
- Polymerase chain reaction (PCR) – this test amplifies genomic DNA from the bacterial species under investigation and so can confirm the presence of *Treponema pallidum* in congenital syphilis and neurosyphilis. This test may be used clinically in the near future.

Treatment for syphilis

Table 2.1: Recommended treatment regimes			
Clinical stage	**Recommended regimen**	**Alternative regimen**	**Clinical notes**
Incubating syphilis/ epidemiological treatment	• Benzathine penicillin 2.4 MU IM single dose. • Doxycycline 100 mg PO two times daily for 14 days. • Azithromycin 1 g PO stat.		
Early (primary/secondary/early latent) syphilis	• Benzathine penicillin 2.4 MU IM single dose. • Procaine penicillin G 600 000 units IM daily for 10 days.	• Doxycycline 100 mg PO two times daily for 14 days. • Azithromycin 2 g PO stat (immediately) or azithromycin 600 mg daily for 10 days. • Erythromycin 500 mg PO four times daily for 14 days. • Ceftriaxone 500 mg IM daily for 10 days. • Amoxicillin 500 mg PO four times daily for 14 days plus probenecid 500 mg PO four times daily for 14 days.	

Clinical stage	Recommended regimen	Alternative regimen	Clinical notes
Late latent, cardiovascular and gummatous syphilis.	• Benzathine penicillin 2.4 MU IM initially and then weekly for two more weeks (three doses in total). • Procaine penicillin 600 000 units IM once daily for 17 days.	• Doxycycline 100 mg PO two times daily for 28 days. • Amoxicillin 2 g PO three times daily plus probenecid 500 mg PO four times daily for 25 days.	Steroid cover should be given when treating cardiovascular syphilis.
Neurosyphilis.	• Procaine penicillin 1.8 MU to 2.4 MU IM once daily plus probenecid 500 mg PO four times daily for 17 days. • Benzylpenicillin 18 MU to 24 MU daily, given as 3 MU to 4 MU IV every four hours for 17 days.	• Doxycycline 200 mg PO two times daily for 28 days. • Amoxicillin 2 g PO three times daily plus probenecid 500 mg PO four times daily for 28 days. • Ceftriaxone 2 g IM once daily for 10 to 14 days.	
Treatment of early syphilis in pregnancy.	• Benzathine penicillin 2.4 MU IM single dose in the first and second trimesters. When maternal treatment is initiated in the third trimester, a second dose of benzathine penicillin 2.4 MU IM should be given after one week (i.e. on day 8). • Procaine penicillin G 600 000 units IM daily for 10 days.	• Amoxicillin 500 mg PO four times daily plus probenecid 500 mg PO four times daily for 14 days. • Ceftriaxone 500 mg IM daily for 10 days. • Erythromycin 500 mg PO four times daily for 14 days or azithromycin 500 mg PO daily for 10 days plus evaluation and treatment of neonates at birth with penicillin.	Management should be in close liaison with obstetric, midwifery and paediatric colleagues. Appropriate follow-up of babies is required.
Treatment of late syphilis in pregnancy.	Manage as in non-pregnant patient but without the use of doxycycline.		
Syphilis treatment in HIV-positive people.	Treatment as appropriate for the stage of infection.		

A note on Jarisch–Herxheimer's reaction

Jarisch–Herxheimer's reaction was first described by Jarish in 1895 and elaborated by Herxheimer in 1902. The reaction was originally observed in patients with syphilis who received mercury treatment and is characterised by transient local and systemic symptoms. The reaction is thought to be caused by the release of toxins from large numbers of infectious organisms as they die off. Four to six hours after starting antisyphilitic treatment, patients may experience headache, chills, nausea, fever, muscle aches and pains, and exacerbation of initial lesions (Fig. 2.35 which may be compared with Fig. 2.16, page 13).

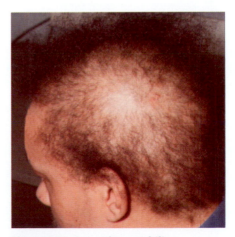

Figure 2.35: Secondary syphilis: exacerbation of alopecia due to Jarisch–Herxheimer's reaction.

Symptoms generally disappear within 24 hours, but some patients will need a short course of steroid therapy.

Patient follow-up

All patients should have serological tests for syphilis 3, 6, 12 and 24 months after diagnosis and treatment. For congenital syphilis, non-treponemal tests should be carried out every 2 to 3 months until a negative result is obtained; for neurosyphilis, cerebrospinal fluid should be examined 6-monthly for 3 years.

Serological tests for syphilis

Following treatment for syphilis, serological tests may be performed to assess response.

Table 2.2: Serological test results expected at each stage of syphilis				
Serological test				
Stage of syphilis	**VDRL[1]**	**TPHA[2]**	**IgM[3]**	**Other**
• Primary, four-weekly after infection	Positive	Positive	Positive	
• Secondary	Positive	Positive	Positive	
• Early latent	Positive	Positive	Positive	
• Late latent	Positive	Positive	Negative	
• Tertiary (late syphilis)	Negative	Positive	Negative	
Neurosyphilis	Positive			Cerebrospinal fluid examination: • white cell count increased. • proline 70.4 mmol/L

[1] VDRL: venereal disease research laboratory test.
[2] TPHA: *Treponema pallidum* haemagglutination test.
[3] Immunoglobulin M antibody test.

Before serology becomes positive, *T. pallidum* can be directly identified by analysing fluid from a primary chancre or aspirated fluid from a regional lymph node.

Serological results and retreatment

If serum titres in serological tests are rising for a treated patient, the patient should be treated again and followed-up as normal.

Chapter 3: Gonorrhoea

History

Gonorrhoea is a sexually transmitted infection. The causative gonococcus bacterium was discovered in 1879 by Albert Ludwig Sigesmund Neisser (1855–1916) at the age of 24, and the species named after him. The organism was subsequently isolated in pure culture in 1885 by Ernst von Bumm.

Causative organism

The causative pathogen, *Neisseria gonorrhoeae*, is a gonococcus bacterium of which there are four types: T1, T2, T3 and T4, each producing colonies of different size, shape and colour in laboratory culture. T1 and T2 are virulent while T3 and T4 are not. Other members of the *Neisseria* genus include pathogenic and non-pathogenic species:

Pathogenic species

- *Neisseria gonorrhoeae (Fig. 3.1).*
- *Neisseria meningitidis.*

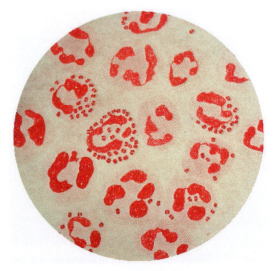

Figure 3.1: Intracellular diplococci: *Neisseria gonorrhoeae.*

Non-pathogenic species

- *Neisseria cinerea.*
- *Neisseria elongata.*
- *Neisseria flavescens.*
- *Neisseria lactamica.*
- *Neisseria mucosa.*
- *Neisseria polysaccharea.*
- *Neisseria sicca.*
- *Neisseria subflava.*
- *Branhamella catarrhalis.*
- *Neisseria bacilliformis.*
- *Neisseria macacae.*

Morphology

Neisseria gonorrhoeae is a gram-negative intracellular diplococcus 0.6 μm to 1.0 μm in diameter, oval to circular in shape, usually seen in pairs (diplococci) with flattened sides at the area of contact. It is often present in polymorphonuclear leucocytes (neutrophils) of the gonorrhoea pustular exudate.

Mode of transmission

- Sexual contact.
- Autoinoculation.
- Mother to foetus (during delivery).

Incubation period

Five to eight days.

Symptoms

Clinical symptoms in male

- Mucopurulent or purulent urethral discharge (Fig. 3.2).
- Urethral discharge.
- Redness and oedema of the urethral meatus.
- Dysuria.

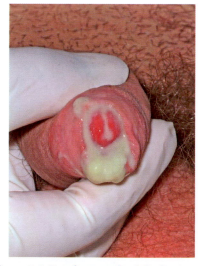

Figure 3.2: Purulent urethral discharge.

Clinical symptoms in female

- Asymptomatic.
- Vaginal discharge.
- Lower abdominal pain.
- Dysuria.
- Vaginal and cervical mucopurulent discharge (Fig. 3.3).

Extragenital symptoms

- Rectal infection.
- Oropharyngeal infection.
- Conjunctival infection (gonococcal conjunctivitis) (Fig. 3.4).

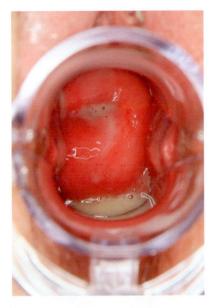

Figure 3.3: Vaginal and cervical mucopurulent discharge.

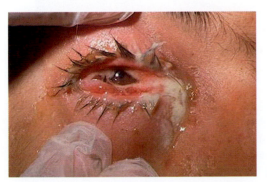

Figure 3.4: Gonococcal conjunctivitis.

Clinical features of rectal infection

Rectal gonorrhoea infection in females is sometimes due to infected vaginal discharge coming into contact with the rectum; alternatively, anal intercourse with an infected male may be the cause (either gender). Rectal infection is usually asymptomatic.

Pharyngeal infection

This is due to oral sex or contact with an infected partner, and is generally asymptomatic.

Ophthalmic infection

Due to autoinoculation from the site of infection (e.g. genitals); conjunctivitis with purulent discharge is the main symptom.

Gonococcal ophthalmia neonatorum (Fig. 3.5) (bilateral conjunctivitis) may occur in newborn children due to an infected mother passing the disease to the child during birth or even in utero. It can be diagnosed within 21 days of birth from appearance of the following symptoms: purulent discharge from the eyes, redness and swelling. Without treatment, the baby can develop corneal ulceration, perforation and ultimately blindness.

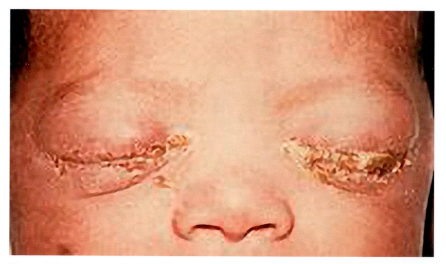

Figure 3.5: Gonococcal ophthalmia neonatorum. (Courtesy of CDC)

Diagnosis

The presence of gram-negative intracellular diplococci bacteria (*Neisseria gonorrhoeae*) can be confirmed by microscopic examination of gram-stained pus from the urethra or endocervical rectum (Fig. 3.6).

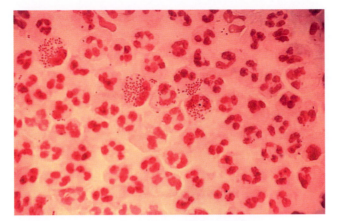

Figure 3.6: Gram-negative intracellular diplococci.

Laboratory tests to confirm diagnosis

- Transport media (Amies' charcoal swab).
- Nucleic acid amplification test (NAAT): polymerase chain reaction (PCR) of urine from male patients and vaginal swab from female patients.
- Real-time PCR: the COBAS 4800 platform qualitatively detects the presence of *Neisseria gonorrhoeae*. The detection of PCR product is monitored by measuring the intensity of fluorescent dyes that are released during the amplification process and comparing with internal controls, measured at a different wavelength. The diagnosis of *N. gonorrhoeae* can be further confirmed by a selective medium called GC CHOC (chocolate agar) which contains a lysed blood supplement and a combination of antibodies that suppress genital tract flora and allow for growth of *N. gonorrhoeae*. This medium is suitable for all swab types (rectal, urethral, cervical and throat). A monoclonal antibody agglutination kit specific for gonorrhoea can also be used to confirm diagnosis.
- Minimal inhibitory concentration (MIC), the lowest concentration of a given antibiotic that inhibits the growth of a specific organism. An MIC test can isolate penicillinase-producing *Neisseria gonorrhoeae* and other resistant organisms of *Neisseria gonorrhoeae*. *Neisseria gonorrhoeae* can be differentiated by sugar fermentation test.

Complications

Local complications in males

- Tysonitis (inflammation of the preputial glands).
- Littritis (inflammation of Littré's gland).
- Cowperitis (inflammation of Cowper's gland).
- Prostatitis (inflammation of the prostate gland).

- Trigonitis (inflammation of the trigone area of the urinary bladder).
- Cystitis (inflammation of the urinary bladder).
- Seminal vesiculitis (inflammation of the seminal vesicles).
- Epididymitis (inflammation of the epididymis).
- Orchitis (inflammation or swelling of the testis).
- Periurethral abscess (Fig. 3.7).
- Proctitis (inflammation of the rectum, usually in homosexual men).
- Urethral strictures (Fig. 3.8).

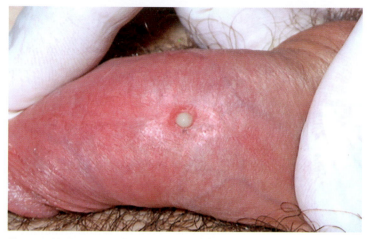

Figure 3.7: Gonococcal periurethral abscess.

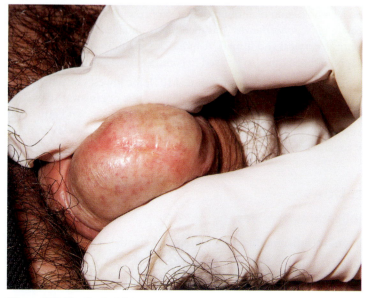

Figure 3.8: Urethral stricture.

Local complications in females

- Skenitis (inflammation of Skene's gland).
- Bartholinitis (inflammation of Bartholin's gland), Bartholin's cyst or abscess (Fig. 3.9).
- Cystitis.
- Pelvic inflammatory disease.
- Infertility.

Systemic complications

- Disseminated gonococcal infection.
  - Skin infection (gonococcal septicaemia) (Fig. 3.10).
  - Arthritis.

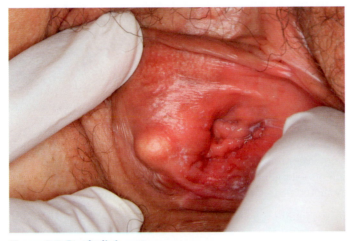

Figure 3.9: Bartholin's cyst.

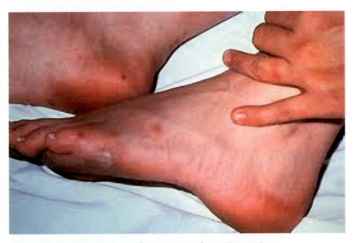

Figure 3.10: Skin lesion of gonococcal septicaemia.

- Endocarditis.
- Meningitis.
- Perihepatitis (Fitz-Hugh–Curtis's syndrome, first described by Arthur Hale Curtis in 1930 and again, independently, by Thomas Fitz-Hugh in 1934). This condition is characterised by friction between the liver and surrounding tissue, fever, abdominal pain and spasm.

Management of Gonorrhoea

Without complications (single doses)

- Ceftriaxone 200 mg intramuscular, first line of treatment.
- Cefixime 400 mg tablet orally.
- Spectinomycin 2 g intramuscular, as alternative therapy.
- Ciprofloxacin 400 mg orally – tablet or liquid suspension.
- Ampicillin 3 g orally in combination with probenecid 1 g orally.

With complications

One of the above drugs can be used (single dose), followed by a course of ciprofloxacin 500 mg two times a day for seven days.

Some gonococcal strains have become resistant to tetracycline and quinolones, so these are generally not recommended. Pharyngeal and rectal gonorrhoea should be treated similarly. If patients with gonococcal infection have a suspected co-infection of chlamydial urethritis, they should be treated with a single dose of azithromycin 1 g oral tablet.

Pregnant women should be treated as above (note that tetracycline and quinolones are contraindicated in pregnancy).

Chapter 4: Urethritis due to Chlamydia trachomatis

Aetiology

Chlamydial urethritis is inflammation of the urethra due to *Chlamydia trachomatis* infection. *C. trachomatis* is a pathogenic bacterium which is dependent on the host's cells to live, and cannot survive outside a living cell. Although *C. trachomatis* can cause eye and respiratory disease, it usually infects the lower urogenital tract, and is the most common sexually transmitted infection (STI).

Incubation period

Generally 1 to 3 weeks after infection.

Symptoms

Chlamydial urethritis may be asymptomatic, but the following symptoms may be present:

- swelling of the urethra.
- pain when urinating – often a burning sensation.
- white or clear discharge from the penis, from the urethral opening (Fig. 4.1).
- vaginal discharge (Fig. 4.2, next page).
- cervical erosion (Fig. 4.3, next page).

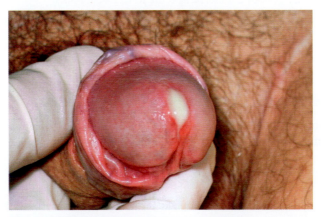

Figure 4.1: Mucoid discharge due to chlamydia.

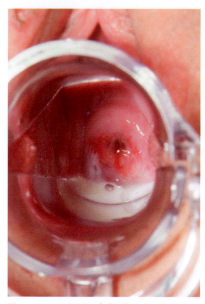

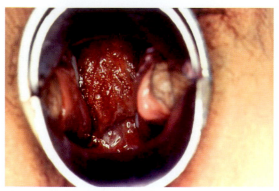

Figure 4.2: Vaginal discharge due to chlamydia.

Figure 4.3: Cervical erosion due to chlamydia infection.

Diagnosis

Urethritis is confirmed by the presence of raised numbers of white blood cells in the urethral discharge under gram staining.

Presence of *C. trachomatis* can be confirmed by several techniques.

- Culture from swab of urethral discharge.
- Urine test.
- Nucleic acid amplification test (NAAT), e.g. polymerase chain reaction (PCR) to identify genomic material specific to *C. trachomatis.*
- All patients with suspected infection should also be tested for gonorrhoea since the symptoms for gonorrhoea may be similar to those for chlamydia, and these diseases often occur together.

Complications

Untreated chlamydial urethritis can lead to different complications in males and females as follows, with some of the complications resembling those from untreated gonococcal infections.

Males

- Epididymitis – *C. trachomatis* infection of the epididymis, causing swelling and testicular pain.

- Reiter's syndrome – reactive arthritis affecting mainly joints below the waist. Usually occurs one to three weeks after the initial chlamydial infection and is often accompanied by conjunctivitis and lesions on the skin and mucous membranes (*see* Chapter 9, page 51).

Females

- Pelvic inflammatory disease (PID) – a serious *C. trachomatis* infection of the reproductive organs including the uterus and fallopian tubes. Scarring and blockage of the fallopian tubes may occur, leading to infertility, ectopic pregnancy and miscarriage (*see* Chapter 6, page 43).
- Mothers may transmit *C. trachomatis* infection to a newborn child, leading to chlamydial pneumonia and bacterial conjunctivitis (ophthalmia neonatorum) in the child.
- Reiter's syndrome (*see* 'Males' section above, and Chapter 9, page 51) – less frequent in females than in males.

Treatment

Antibiotics are used to manage chlamydial urethritis, with specific treatment depending on whether the condition is uncomplicated or complicated.

Uncomplicated chlamydial urethritis

- Azithromycin 1 g orally, single dose.
- Doxycycline 100 mg orally two times daily for seven days.
- Alternatively:
  - erythromycin base 500 mg orally four times per day for seven days.
  - erythromycin ethylsuccinate 800 mg orally four times per day for seven days.
  - ofloxacin 300 mg two times daily for seven days.
  - levofloxacin 500 mg once daily for seven days.

Complicated chlamydial urethritis

- PID:
  - ofloxacin 400 mg orally two times daily for 14 days.
  - levofloxacin 500 mg orally once daily for 14 days; may be administered in combination with metronidazole 500 mg orally two times daily for 14 days.
  - cefotetan 2 g intravenous every 12 hours, administered in combination with doxycycline 100 mg orally (or intravenous) every 12 hours, for 14 days.
  - cefoxitin 2 g intravenous every six hours, administered in combination with doxycycline 100 mg orally (or intravenous) every 12 hours, for 14 days.

- Pregnancy – doxycycline and ofloxacin are contraindicated during pregnancy so the treatments of choice are:
  - erythromycin base 500 mg orally four times per day for seven days.
  - amoxicillin 500 mg orally three times per day for seven days.
  - erythromycin ethylsuccinate 400 mg four times per day for 14 days.
  - azithromycin 1 g orally, single dose.
- Reiter's syndrome – the antibiotic therapies given above for uncomplicated chlamydial urethritis will address the underlying cause of Reiter's syndrome. The symptoms of joint pain can be treated with non-steroidal anti-inflammatory drugs (NSAIDs), or in severe cases, corticosteroid injections.
- Ophthalmia neonatorum in newborn children:
  - erythromycin base 50 mg/kg/day orally, administered as 12.5 mg four times per day, for 14 days.
  - erythromycin ethylsuccinate 50 mg/kg/day orally for 14 days, administered as above.
- Chlamydial pneumonia:
  - erythromycin base 50 mg/kg/day orally, administered as 12.5 mg four times per day, for 14 days.
  - erythromycin ethylsuccinate 50 mg/kg/day orally for 14 days, administered as above.

For ophthalmia neonatorum and chlamydial pneumonia, a second course of antibiotics may be necessary.

To prevent passing the infection to others, sexual partners should also be treated, even if they are asymptomatic.

Chapter 5: Non-specific urethritis

Aetiology

Non-specific urethritis is inflammation of the urethra, due to an unknown cause but identified as *not* being due to a gonococcal infection (this condition is therefore also referred to as non-gonococcal urethritis). Other possible causes of non-specific urethritis include sexually transmitted infections with *Chlamydia trachomatis*, *Trichomonas vaginalis* (a protozoan parasite), *Mycoplasma genitalium* (a bacterium which often co-infects with other bacterial species) and genital *Herpes simplex virus* (a virus which also causes cold sores). Non-specific urethritis is most frequently diagnosed in males, as the disease in females is often asymptomatic. However, if untreated, non-specific urethritis due to *chlamydia* or *mycoplasma* may lead to pelvic inflammatory disease (*see* Chapter 6, page 43) in women.

Incubation period – several weeks to several months following an initial infection.

Symptoms

Many cases of non-specific urethritis are asymptomatic, but when symptoms do present they may be different in males and females.

Males

- Discharge from the urethra – white or opaque in appearance (Fig. 5.1).
- Dysuria – pain or burning sensation when passing urine.
- A need to urinate frequently.

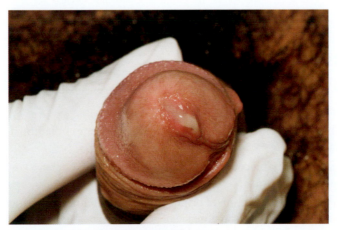

Figure 5.1: Mucoid urethral discharge.

Females

- Vaginal discharge (Fig. 5.2).
- Fever.
- Lower abdominal pain.
- Deep pelvic pain during sexual intercourse.
- Bleeding after intercourse and between menstruation.

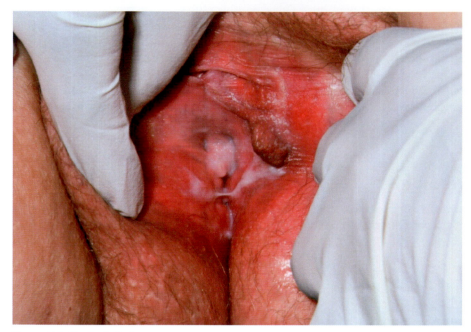

Figure 5.2: Vaginal discharge.

Diagnosis

Tests are used to confirm urethritis and rule out gonococcal and chlamydia infections.

- Microscopic examination of urethral swab:
  - high white blood cell count (leucocytes) indicates inflammation (Figs. 5.3 and 5.4).
  - absence of gonococcal or *Chlamydia trachomatis* bacteria confirm non-specific urethritis.
- Urine test – examination of urine sample (four hours after the patient last passed urine) to confirm absence of gonococcal or *Chlamydia trachomatis* bacteria and possibly identify other causative species.

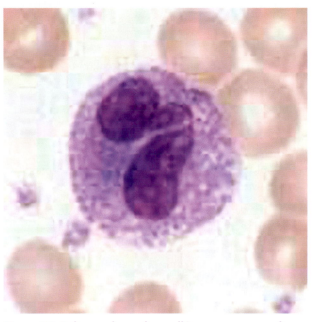

Figure 5.3: Polymorphonuclear cell in non-gonococcal urethritis.

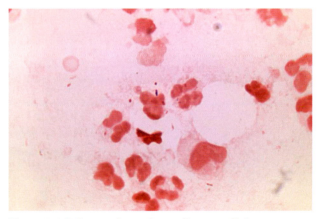

Figure 5.4: Polymorphonuclear cells: pus cells in non-gonococcal urethritis.

Complications

- Persistent urethritis – recurrence of symptoms even after treatments.
- Reiter's syndrome – reactive arthritis; an autoimmune response to infection causing joint pain, recurrent urethritis and conjunctivitis (*see* Chapter 9, page 51).
- Epididymitis and orchitis (epididymo-orchitis) – in males: inflammation of the epididymis and testis, respectively.

Treatment

Uncomplicated non-specific urethritis

Antibiotics are the standard therapy for non-gonococcal, non-specific urethritis.

- Azithromycin 1 g orally, single dose.
- Doxycycline 200 mg orally, two times per day for 10 days.

Complicated non-specific urethritis

The above treatment should be administered, with additional treatment (where appropriate) for complications as follows:

Reiter's syndrome can be treated with NSAIDs or corticosteroid therapy (systemic or injections into the affected sacroiliac joints) to reduce inflammation and pain (*see* Chapter 9, page 51).

Epididymo-orchitis is treated with NSAIDs for the inflammation plus antibiotics for any suspected underlying bacterial infection.

- Ceftriaxone 250 mg intramuscular single dose, plus doxycycline 100 mg orally two times per day for 10 to 14 days.
- Alternatives:
  - ofloxacin 200 mg orally two times per day for 14 days.
  - ciprofloxacin 500 mg orally two times per day for 10 days.

It is recommended that all sexual partners are also treated for non-specific urethritis as it can be transmitted during sexual intercourse.

Chapter 6: Pelvic inflammatory disease

Aetiology

Pelvic inflammatory disease (PID) is inflammation of the female upper reproductive tract caused by bacterial infection, often introduced during sexual intercourse. The uterus, fallopian tubes and ovaries are affected, usually the result of infection in the vagina or cervix spreading upwards. PID may be caused by a number of bacterial species, with the STIs chlamydia and gonorrhoea being the most frequent. Sexually active women between the ages of 16 and 25 years are most often affected, but it can occur in any sexually active woman.

Incubation period

The occurrence of PID following an STI infection is highly variable and may be from a few days to six months after initial vaginal/cervical infection.

Symptoms

Some cases are asymptomatic; otherwise any of the following symptoms may be present:

- lower abdominal pain.
- pelvic pain during sexual intercourse.
- dysuria – pain when passing urine.
- rectal pain.
- vaginal discharge – may be yellow or green in colour.
- bleeding after intercourse.
- fever.
- vomiting.

Diagnosis

PID is characterised by salpingitis (inflammation of the fallopian tubes), oophoritis (inflammation of the ovaries), parametritis (inflammation of the tissue around the uterus – the parametrium) and endometritis (inflammation of the uterus lining – the endometrium). No single test can diagnose PID: diagnosis is based on a combination of clinical symptoms, laboratory tests and imaging tests.

- Clinical symptoms.
- Laboratory tests:
  - culture from vaginal swab – to confirm presence of causative bacterial species (not always positive in PID cases).
  - white blood cell count – higher than $10.5 \times 10^9/L$ indicates inflammation due to infection.
  - red blood cell sedimentation rate (ESR) test – higher than 15 mm per hour.
  - pregnancy test (urine and blood test for human chorionic gonadotropin – hCG), to exclude ectopic pregnancy.
- Imaging tests:
  - ultrasound scan – may be negative for mild cases of PID.
  - laparoscopy – internal endoscopic examination of the reproductive organs to identify inflammation; most useful in suspected severe cases.

Complications

- Recurrence of PID – more than one episode is associated with a greater chance of recurrence.
- Abscesses – the infection can cause abscesses of the ovaries or fallopian tubes which can be serious if untreated.
- Scarring and blockage of the fallopian tubes – may lead to ectopic pregnancy (growth of the foetus outside the uterus – usually in the fallopian tubes).
- Infertility – blockage of the fallopian tubes by scar tissue may make natural conception impossible; in such cases, in vitro fertilisation (IVF) should be considered by women wishing to become pregnant.

Treatment

Suspected PID should be diagnosed and treated promptly, as untreated PID is likely to result in potentially serious complications.

- Antibiotics – two are often prescribed in combination as more than one bacterial species may be causative.
  - Ofloxacin – 400 mg orally two times per day for 10 to 14 days.
  - Metronidazole – 500 mg orally two times per day for 14 days.
  - Ceftriaxone – 500 mg intramuscular single dose for mild PID, or 1 g to 2 g intravenous or intramuscular once daily for 14 days for severe cases. Use with lidocaine, intramuscular stat (immediate) single dose.
  - Doxycycline – 100 mg orally or intravenous two times per day for 14 days, in combination with another antibiotic.

- Surgery
  - Laparoscopy – keyhole surgery to remove scar tissue or unblock fallopian tubes; can lead to further scarring.
  - Salpingectomy – removal of a fallopian tube to stop the spread of infection; only for severe cases as removal of both fallopian tubes results in infertility.

Ectopic pregnancy can be treated with a single dose of methotrexate 50 g/m^2 (body surface area) intramuscular if caught early and the fallopian tube has not ruptured. In other cases, surgery is required:

- Salpingostomy – removal of the pregnancy.
- Salpingectomy – removal of a fallopian tube.
- Fimbrial expression – pushing the pregnancy out of the fallopian tube without incision.

All patients with PID should be counselled on the causes of the disease and the importance of safe sexual practice.

Chapter 7: Prostatitis

Aetiology

Prostatitis is inflammation of the prostate gland and may be caused by bacterial infection. There are four types of prostatitis:

- acute bacterial prostatitis.
- chronic bacterial prostatitis.
- chronic non-bacterial prostatitis.
- asymptomatic inflammatory prostatitis.

The causes of bacterial prostatitis are usually the bacteria *E. coli*, klebsiella and proteus. The most common form of prostatitis is chronic non-bacterial. The cause of this type is unknown and is also referred to as 'chronic pelvic pain syndrome'. Acute bacterial prostatitis may be transmitted via sexual contact so is regarded as a sexually transmitted infection (STI). Prostatitis can occur in males at any age.

Symptoms

Acute bacterial prostatitis

- fever.
- shivering.
- pelvic or genital pain.
- dysuria – pain or difficulty passing urine (intermittent flow).
- pain when ejaculating.

Chronic prostatitis – bacterial and non-bacterial

May be asymptomatic, but when present, symptoms are similar to those for acute bacterial prostatitis, although less painful. Other symptoms may include:

- fatigue.
- joint or muscle pain.

Asymptomatic chronic prostatitis

There are no symptoms – a high white blood cell count is sometimes seen during routine testing.

Diagnosis

- Clinical presentation and history.
- Digital rectal examination (DRE) – to feel if the prostate is tender and inflamed.
- Urine analysis – to identify bacterial infections and measure white cell count.
- Culture from urine sample – to isolate and identify any bacterial species present.
- Prostate specific antigen test from blood sample – raised level indicates prostate inflammation.

Complications

Acute bacterial prostatitis can result in permanent prostate damage if not treated promptly. Chronic bacterial prostatitis may spread to the ureters, kidneys, bladder or urethra if not treated.

Treatment

Acute bacterial prostatitis

- Ciprofloxacin 500 mg orally two times per day for 28 days.
- Doxycycline 100 mg orally two times per day for 28 days.
- Non-steroidal anti-inflammatory drugs (NSAIDs) for symptomatic pain relief.

Chronic bacterial prostatitis

- Oral antibiotics – as for acute bacterial prostatitis – in combination with an alpha blocker to relax the bladder muscle and improve urinary problems, e.g. alfuzosin 10 mg orally, once daily.
- Non-steroidal anti-inflammatory drugs (NSAIDs) for symptomatic pain relief.

Chronic non-bacterial prostatitis

- Alpha blocker to relax the bladder muscle, e.g. alfuzosin 10 mg orally, once daily for four to eight weeks.
- Non-steroidal anti-inflammatory drugs (NSAIDs) for symptomatic pain relief.

Asymptomatic chronic prostatitis

No treatment required.

Chapter 8: Epididymitis and epididymo-orchitis

Aetiology

Epididymo-orchitis is inflammation and swelling of the epididymis and testis (epididymitis – inflammation of epididymis; orchitis – inflammation of testis) due to infection or trauma. The condition may occur unilaterally or bilaterally. The epididymis is a tightly coiled tube on the posterior side of each testis that transports spermatozoa to the vas deferens. The condition usually occurs in young men.

Epididymitis may be acute or chronic. Infection usually starts in the epididymus and secondarily affects the testis, resulting in epididymo-orchitis.

There are many possible causes of acute epididymitis, including bacterial infections, viral infections and trauma, as follows:

- bacterial species including *E. coli*, streptococcus and staphylococcus.
- non-gonococcal urethritis.
- gonococcal epididymitis.
- retrograde passage of infected urine into the vas deferens.
- trauma.
- tuberculosis.
- mumps.
- lymphogranuloma venereum – an STI caused by *Chlamydia trachomatis*.
- chronic prostatitis.
- *Brucella* spp. – coccobacilli which may be transmitted via sexual contact.
- Behçet's disease.
- sarcoidosis.

Symptoms

- Pain in testis.
- Swelling of the testis.
- Scrotum becomes red and inflamed (Fig. 8.1).
- Haematospermia – blood in the semen.
- Pyrexia.

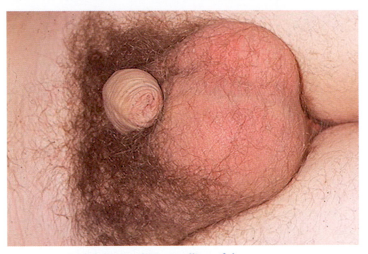

Figure 8.1: Epididymo-orchitis: swelling of the scrotum.

Diagnosis

- Full STI screening – including gonorrhoea and *Chlamydia trachomatis*.
- Urine examination (midstream sample of urine – MSSU).
- Ultrasound of scrotum and testis – increased vascularity of the testis and the tail of the epididymis suggests epididymo-orchitis (Fig. 8.2).

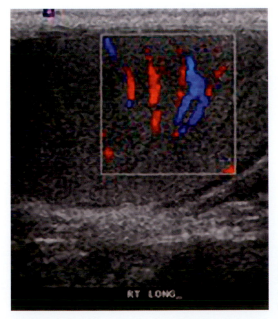

Figure 8.2: Ultrasound showing increased vascularity of tail of epididymis and testis: suggestive of epididymo-orchitis.

Complications

- Abscess – requires surgical attention.
- Reduced fertility or infertility.
- Chronic epididymo-orchitis may develop.

Treatment

Treatment is in accordance with the nature of the infection.

- Chlamydia and gonorrhoea – doxycycline tablets 100 mg two times per day for 14 days in combination with either cefixime 400 mg stat (immediate) oral dose, or ceftriaxone 500 mg intramuscular, single dose.
- Ofloxacin 200 mg orally two times per day for 14 days.
- Ciprofloxacin 500 mg orally two times per day for 14 days.
- Scrotal support.
- Analgesics – NSAIDs.

Chapter 9: Reiter's syndrome

History

Reiter's syndrome, also called reactive arthritis, is a condition caused by an immunological reaction to infection. It was first described in 1916 by Hans Reiter and again, independently, in the same year by Fiessinger and Leroy who called the condition oculo-urethro-synovial syndrome. Reiter's syndrome is associated with infection by several pathogenic bacterial species such as *Shigella*, *Salmonella* and *Campylobacter*, and the sexually transmitted infection *Chlamydia trachomatis*, which causes genito-urinary infections.

Aetiology

Reiter's syndrome usually develops two to six weeks after non-gonococcal urethritis caused by *Chlamydia trachomatis* infection. The disease is caused by a systemic and intrasynovial autoimmune response to the infection.

Symptoms

There is a classic triad of conditions comprising Reiter's syndrome:

- urethritis.
- conjunctivitis.
- arthritis.

Urethritis

This may be asymptomatic but the following symptoms may be present:

- swelling of the urethra.
- dysuria – pain when urinating, often a burning sensation.
- white or clear discharge from the penis in males, or from the urethral opening in females during pelvic examination.

Conjunctivitis

- Reddening of the whites of the eyes.
- Painful or burning sensation in the eyes.
- Watery eyes.

Arthritis

- Pain and swelling of weight-bearing joints, but other joints may also be involved.
- Lower back pain.
- Swelling and tenderness of the Achilles tendon.

Other symptoms of Reiter's syndrome

- Keratoderma blennorrhagica – scaly rash on the palms and soles (Fig. 9.1).
- Circinate balanitis (in males) – inflammation of the skin on the glans penis, often a white, scaly, dermatitis (Fig. 9.2).
- Thick and crumbly nails.
- Aortitis – causes aortic regurgitation in rare cases.

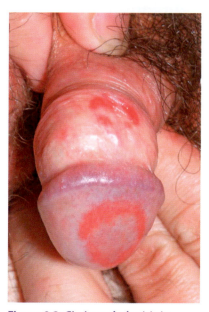

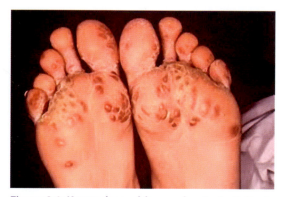

Figure 9.1: Keratoderma blennorrhagica in Reiter's syndrome. (Courtesy Dr N Khanna and Mehta Publishing House)

Figure 9.2: Circinate balanitis in Reiter's syndrome.

Diagnosis

Diagnosis of Reiter's syndrome is confirmed using laboratory and imaging tests. There is a fusion of both SI joints, and visible lower facet joints suggests Reiter's syndrome.

Laboratory

- Erythrocyte sedimentation rate (ESR) test – indicates inflammation if raised, but is not specific.
- C-reactive protein (CRP) test – indicates inflammation if raised; levels return to normal following successful treatment.
- Microscopic examination of synovial fluid – raised white blood cell count and presence of specific bacterial antigens.
- Culture from urethral discharge – to identify chlamydia.
- Perform HLAB-27 test.

Imaging tests

- Radiography – in advanced Reiter's syndrome, calcaneal spurs are seen on the feet, and bone proliferation with areas of erosion is present in the hands and feet. Other possible signs include sacroiliitis of the spine, with non-marginal syndesmophytes in the thoracolumbar region (Fig. 9.3).
- Magnetic resonance imaging (MRI) – changes to the sacroiliac joints can be observed.

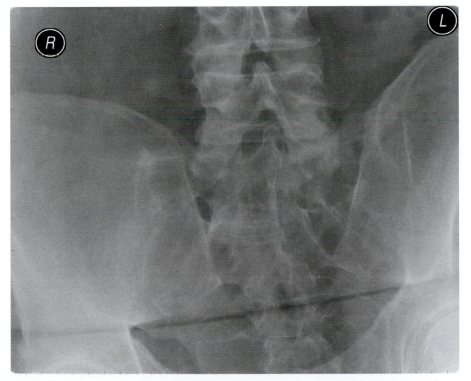

Figure 9.3: Reactive arthritis due to Reiter's syndrome. (Courtesy of Dr Deep Chand)

Complications

Long-term untreated Reiter's syndrome may result in the following complications:

- aortic insufficiency (also referred to as aortic regurgitation) – the aortic valve of the heart fails to close properly, causing blood from the aorta to flow back into the left ventricle.
- cardiac arrhythmia – abnormal rhythm of the heart causing less efficient pumping.
- uveitis – inflammation of the middle layer of the eye comprising the iris, ciliary body and choroid.

Treatment

Symptom relief

- Non-steroidal anti-inflammatory drugs – these reduce inflammation and relieve pain.
- Alternative: systemic corticosteroid therapy – prednisone 0.5–1 mg/kg/day (depending on severity of symptoms) and adjusted on an individual basis.
- Corticosteroid injections into the affected sacroiliac joints – these reduce swelling and joint pain.
- Disease-modifying antirheumatic drugs (DMARDs) – for patients not responding to NSAIDs or corticosteroids. DMARDs prevent the immune system attacking healthy tissue, thus removing the mechanism of Reiter's disease. They may take four to six months to work so adherence to the medication is very important and should be stressed to patients.

Antimicrobials

The underlying *Chlamydia trachomatis* infection should be treated with antibiotics.

- Azithromycin 1 g orally, single dose.
- Doxycycline 100 mg orally two times daily for seven days.
- Alternatively:
  - erythromycin base 500 mg orally four times per day for seven days.
  - erythromycin ethylsuccinate 800 mg orally four times per day for seven days.
  - ofloxacin 300 mg two times daily for seven days.
  - levofloxacin 500 mg once daily for seven days.

Complications

- Aortic insufficiency can be treated with vasodilators and, in severe cases, valve surgery.

- Cardiac arrhythmia may be treated with beta blockers or antiarrhythmic drugs (e.g. flecainide or amiodarone), or in severe cases, surgery.
- Uveitis is treated with steroid eye-drops (e.g. prednisone acetate), often in combination with mydriatic eye-drops (pupil dilators, e.g. atropine). Severe cases may require oral steroids (e.g. prednisolone), a periocular steroid injection, or treatment with an immunosuppressant drug (cyclosporin or methotrexate).

Chapter 10: Bacterial vaginosis

Aetiology

Bacterial vaginosis is a common condition affecting the vagina, in which the balance of normally occurring bacteria becomes altered resulting in abnormal discharge. The condition is often associated with an increase in vaginal pH, making it more alkaline (pH 4.5 to 7.0), which is due to a decrease in lactobacilli – bacteria naturally present in the vagina which produce lactic acid – allowing other bacterial species to overgrow, including *Gardnerella vaginalis*, *Mycoplasma hominis* and species of *Prevotella* and *Mobiluncus*. It is not clear why the bacterial balance of the vagina changes but several factors may be involved, including:

- sexual activity – sexually active females are more prone to bacterial vaginitis.
- smoking.
- presence of intrauterine device (IUD).
- perfumed or antibacterial bath products – the vagina may be affected during douching.

Symptoms

Many cases of bacterial vaginosis are asymptomatic. If symptoms present, they may be as follows:

- strong, fishy, odour to the vagina – particularly after sexual intercourse.
- grey or white vaginal discharge.
- thin and watery vaginal discharge (Fig. 10.1).

Diagnosis

- Clinical presentation.
- The Amsel criteria – diagnosis is confirmed if at least three of the following four criteria are positive:
  - thin, white, vaginal discharge.
  - specific cells on microscopic examination of smear.

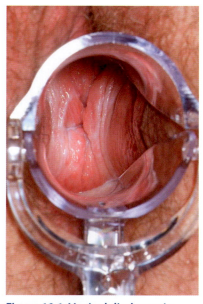

Figure 10.1: Vaginal discharge in bacterial vaginosis.

- – vaginal fluid pH higher than 4.5.
- – fishy odour when alkali added to vaginal fluid.
- Microscopic examination of gram-stained vaginal smear to identify bacterial species levels according to the Hay/Ison criteria (clue cells) (Fig. 10.2).
  - – Grade 1 (normal): lactobacilli are most numerous.
  - – Grade 2 (intermediate): mixed bacterial species with some lactobacilli present but *Gardnerella* or *Mobiluncus* species also present.
  - – Grade 3 (bacterial vaginosis): mostly *Gardnerella* and/or *Mobiluncus* species with few or no lactobacilli present.

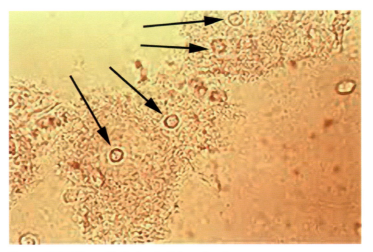

Figure 10.2: Clue cells in bacterial vaginosis.

Complications

Women with bacterial vaginosis may be at greater risk of the following conditions:

- pelvic inflammatory disease (*see* Chapter 6, page 43).
- sexually transmitted infections – including herpes, gonorrhoea and chlamydia.

Pregnant women may be more likely to miscarry late in the pregnancy or undergo premature delivery, and suffer postpartum endometriosis (inflammation of the uterus lining).

Treatment

Antibiotics are the standard treatment for bacterial vaginosis:

- Metronidazole 400 mg orally two times per day for five to seven days (alcohol should be avoided) or alternatively metronidazole 2 g orally, single dose.

- Metronidazole 0.75% gel – applied intravaginally once daily for five days.
- Clindamycin 300 mg orally two times per day for seven days.
- Clindamycin 2% cream – applied intravaginally once daily for seven days.
- Tinidazole 2 g orally, single dose (alcohol should be avoided).

Douching with scented and antiseptic soaps or gels should be avoided. Clindamycin 2% cream should be used for women allergic to metronidazole and those breastfeeding.

Chapter 11: Trichomoniasis

History

Trichomoniasis is a parasitic infection of the vagina and urethra in females, and the urethra and, rarely, the prostate gland in males. The causative organism, *Trichomonas vaginalis,* was first recorded in the literature in 1836 by Alfred Donné, and given its present taxonomic name by Ehrenberg. This parasite was identified and classified on the basis of its morphology by Procaccini between 1930 and 1939. Trichomoniasis is the most common sexually transmitted infection (STI) worldwide.

Causative organism

Trichomonas vaginalis is an anaerobic parasite. It is pear- or diamond-shaped and approximately 10 μm to 23 μm long with five flagella (Fig. 11.1): four to provide motility and one to act as a rudder. In females, the parasite adheres to the vaginal wall and produces tendrils that penetrate the vaginal tissue, where it may remain for two years or more.

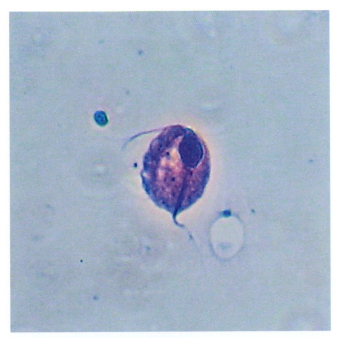

Figure 11.1: *Trichomonas vaginalis.*

Incubation period

Generally 5 to 28 days after exposure.

Mode of transmission

- Vaginal sex (the vast majority of cases).
- Contaminated objects (e.g. sex toys, toilet seats).
- Infected mother to newborn child during childbirth.

Symptoms

Symptoms are often different in males and females, with many cases remaining asymptomatic for several months, particularly in males.

Females

- Vaginal discharge – it may be frothy, yellow or green in colour and have a 'fishy' odour.
- Abdominal discomfort.
- 'Strawberry cervix' – due to tiny haemorrhages caused by *T. vaginalis* (Fig. 11.2).

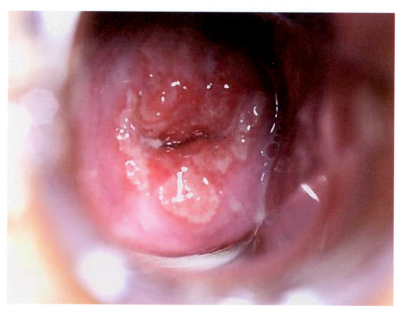

Figure 11.2: Strawberry cervix in trichomoniasis.

- Urethral irritation – possible pain when passing urine.
- Vaginitis – inflammation of the vagina and vulva, causing soreness, itchiness and swelling of the genitals, particularly the labia majora, labia minora and perineum.
- Pain during sexual intercourse.

Males

- Urethral irritation – itching sensation and possible pain when passing urine or after ejaculation.
- Watery discharge from the penis.

Males are generally asymptomatic and are therefore carriers who pass the infection on to their sexual partners.

Diagnosis

- Clinical presentation – inflammation of the genitals and vaginal lining.
- Microscopic examination of vaginal discharge – under dark-field microscopy, characteristic movement of *Trichomonas vaginalis* parasites can confirm diagnosis.
- Gram-stained smear from vaginal swab – the parasite can be observed and identified.
- Urine analysis – motile parasites may be visible under the microscope.
- Laboratory smear from vaginal swab sent in Amies' or Stuart's transport media can be used for diagnosis.

Complications

- During pregnancy – trichomoniasis can cause premature labour and delivery, with low birth weight of the newborn.
- Weakening of the cervix mucous barrier – this increases the risk of other infections of the reproductive organs.
- Non-gonococcal urethritis.
- PID – trichomoniasis is a risk factor.
- Bartholinitis – inflammation of Bartholin's glands near the vaginal opening.
- Drug-resistant parasites can be problematic and contribute to the social STI problem.

Treatment

- Metronidazole is approved to use in pregnancy.
- Metronidazole 400–500 mg orally two times per day for five to seven days.
- Metronidazole 2 g orally, single dose stat (immediately).

The following regimens can be used for patients with metronidazole-resistant infection:

- Increased oral metronidazole 400 mg three times daily for 7 to 10 days, together with oral erythromycin 250 mg four times daily for 5 to 7 days or oral amoxicillin 250 mg three times daily for 5 to 7 days (note that amoxicillin is contraindicated in pregnancy).
- Increased dose of intravenous metronidazole up to 3 g to 3.5 g daily for 14 days together with either amoxicillin or erythromycin for 14 days.
- Acetarsol pessary 500 mg daily for 10 days.
- Paromomycin sulphate pessary 250 mg two times per day for 14 days.
- Nonoxynol[9] pessaries for longer duration (up to three months).

Sexual partners should also be treated with metronidazole 400 mg two times per day for five days. The patient and partner should abstain from sexual intercourse until both are free of infection. Full STI screening is advisable to detect any co-infection such as HIV or *Neisseria gonorrhoeae*.

Chapter 12: Genital candidiasis

Aetiology

Candidiasis is a yeast fungal infection which can affect any part of the body, particularly warm, moist areas such as the vagina, mouth and armpits. Candida is always present on the body and certain physiological factors cause the fungus to flourish and cause infection. There are more than 150 species of candida including:

- *Candida albicans.*
- *Candida tropicalis.*
- *Candida glabrata.*
- *Candida krusei.*
- *Candida parapsilosis.*
- *Candida dubliniensis.*
- *Candida lusitaniae.*

The most common infection is *Candida albicans*, first described in 1923 by Christine Berkhout. Candida – also referred to as moniliasis or 'thrush' – is the most frequent cause of vaginitis. In males candida can cause candida balanitis and candida balanoposthitis.

Predisposing factors

- Sexual contact with an infected partner (hypothetical).
- Diabetes mellitus.
- Hormonal changes – including menstruation, pregnancy and use of oral contraceptives.
- Hormone replacement therapy (oestrogens).
- Presence of semen.
- Immune deficiency.
- Long-term steroid therapy.
- Chemotherapy.
- Long-term antibiotics (in a few documented cases).

Site of involvement

Candida may affect any external part of the body, but particularly warm, moist, areas as follows:

- vagina – candida in the vagina is often called thrush.
- penis – glans and prepuce.
- mouth – common in babies; usually called oral candidiasis or oral thrush.
- armpits.
- groin – especially where pubic hair grows.
- under breasts.
- skin folds.
- nail beds.

Symptoms

Vaginal candidiasis

- Thick, white, discharge – resembles cottage cheese (Fig. 12.1).
- Itching and irritation of the vagina and vulva.
- Dysuria – burning sensation when passing urine.

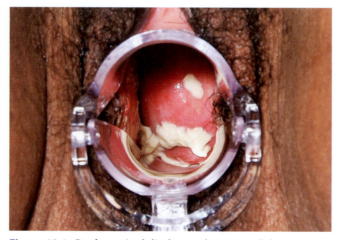

Figure 12.1: Curdy vaginal discharge due to candida.

Candida balanitis/balanoposthitis

- Lesion on the glans penis or inner prepuce – lesion is moist, macular and erythematous (Figs. 12.2 and 12.3).
- Ulceration and discolouration.

Oral candidiasis

- White film coating the tongue, cheeks or roof of the mouth (Fig. 12.4).
- Bleeding of the affected area when the white film is disturbed.

Skin infections of candida

- Flat, red, rash with distinct edges (Fig. 12.5).
- Itching or pain in the affected area.

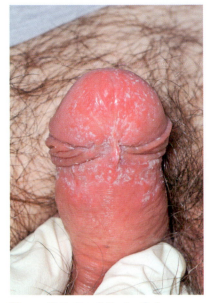

Figure 12.2: Candidiasis of glans penis.

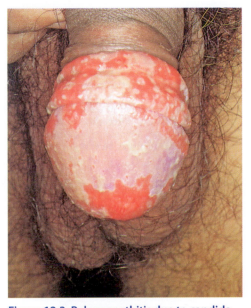

Figure 12.3: Balanoposthitis due to candida. (Courtesy Dr N Khanna and Mehta Publishing House)

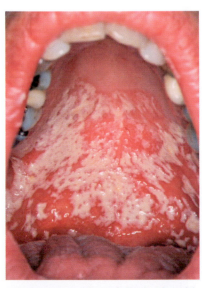

Figure 12.4: Oral candidiasis (thrush).

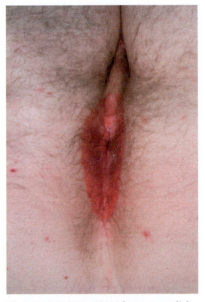

Figure 12.5: Intertrigo due to candida.

Nail bed

- Whitening or yellowing of the nail bed.
- Swelling.
- Loosening of the nail from the nail bed.

Diagnosis

- Clinical presentation – for oral and skin infections.
- Gynaecological examination – for vaginal candidiasis.
- Gram-stained vaginal smear for microscopic examination – microscopic pseudohyphae and spores can be seen (Fig. 12.6).
- Laboratory culture (Amies' Sabouraud media).
- Examination of blood sample – for suspected systemic infection.
- Urethral sample for analysis – for suspected urinary tract infection.

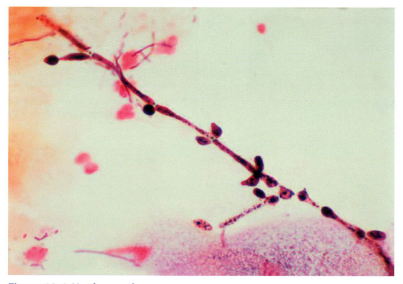

Figure 12.6: Hyphae and spores.

Complications

In people with a compromised immune system, such as those with AIDS or receiving organ antirejection treatment, candida can spread systemically with very serious consequences and is potentially fatal. The most commonly affected organs are the brain, eyes, heart and kidneys. Other complications in this population include:

- oesophagitis – inflammation of the oesophagus.
- candida infection in the stomach.

- ulcers in the gastrointestinal system – can make eating and drinking very painful.
- phimosis due to candida (Fig. 12.7).

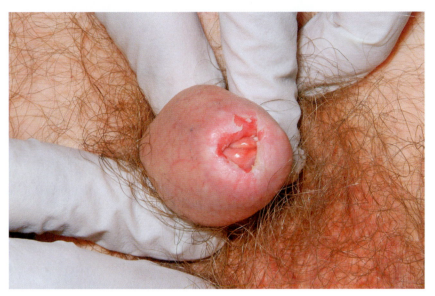

Figure 12.7: Phimosis due to candida.

Treatment

Local application

- Clotrimazole cream and pessary 500 mg, single dose.
- Econazole pessary 150 mg, single dose.
- Miconazole cream and pessary 100 mg daily for 14 days.

The antifungal drug nystatin is available as a pessary and as cream and can be applied for 14 days. Some local application creams are available in combination with hydrocortisone, also available for local application.

Oral therapy

- Fluconazole 150 mg single dose.

Recurrent or chronic balanoposthitis or vaginal candidiasis

Tab fluconazole 100 mg orally stat or 50 mg once daily for 14 days. Intravenous infusion of flucytosine and amphotericin can be used in cases where the infection is resistant to other drugs, and for systemic candida infection. Partners also require treatment to prevent recurrent or chronic candidiasis. Circumcision is indicated in phimosis due to chronic balanoposthitis.

Chapter 13: Tropical genital and sexually acquired infections

13.1: Chancroid

History

Chancroid, also known as 'soft chancre' (not to be confused with syphilitic chancre) and genital ulcer disease (GUD), is a highly contagious sexually transmitted infection caused by the bacterium *Haemophilus ducreyi*. This pathogen was first described by Auguste Ducrey in 1889 and is common in poor areas including Africa, South Asia and the Caribbean.

Causative organism

Haemophilus ducreyi is a short gram-negative coccobacillus (Fig. 13.1.1) – a rod-shaped bacterium which cannot live outside its human host. The organism produces a toxin that contributes to the cause of the characteristic ulcers and delays healing.

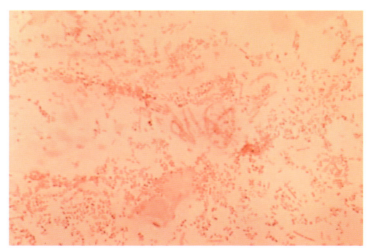

Figure 13.1.1: *Haemophilus ducreyi* of chancroid. (Courtesy of CDC)

Incubation period

This is of short duration, approximately two to seven days.

Symptoms

The initial lesion is usually papular, which progresses to pustular and ultimately ulcerates. Ulcers appear to have a greyish membranous base. Autoinoculation results in multiple lesions at various sites and of different types (Figs. 13.1.2 and 13.1.3).

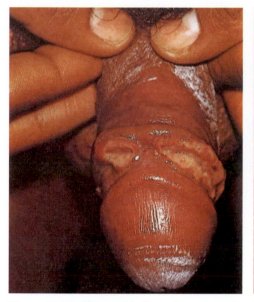

Figure 13.1.2: Chancroid: dirty, deep necrotic ulcer. (Courtesy Dr N Khanna and Mehta Publishing House)

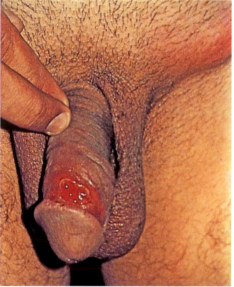

Figure 13.1.3: Chancroid with inflammatory bubo inguinal lymphadenopathy. (Courtesy Dr N Khanna and Mehta Publishing House)

Types of lesion

- Follicular.
- Transient.
- Papular.
- Large ulcer (multiple ulcers).
- Necrotic lesion.

Inguinal lymphadenopathy (swollen lymph nodes in the groin) may also be present.

Sites of involvement

Genital region

- Males.
  - preputial opening.
  - penis shaft.

  - – mucous membranes.
  - – pubic area.
  - – external urinary meatus (urethral opening).
  - – perianal area.
  - – scrotum.
  - – extragenital – due to autoinoculation.
- Females.
  - – fourchette.
  - – labia minora.
  - – vaginal area.

Extragenital sites (by autoinoculation)

- Males.
  - – leg.
  - – foot.
  - – abdomen.
  - – mouth.
- Females.
  - – breast.
  - – lip.
  - – thigh.

Diagnosis

- Direct microscopic examination of gram-stained smear from ulcer – gram-negative bacilli in chain formations may be observed, but are not definitive.
- Culture from ulcer swab (blood-enriched media is necessary for the growth of this species).
- Biopsy – reveals neutrophils, red blood cells and necrotic tissue.
- Tests for syphilis and herpes simplex should be carried out in order to exclude them from the diagnosis.

False positives

Other bacilli species may be present in ulcers, so direct examination should not be the only diagnostic method used.

Complications

- Inguinal abscess – infected and inflamed lymph nodes in the groin (referred to as a bubo).

- Phimosis – constriction of the foreskin due to scar tissue formation.
- Urethral stricture.

Treatment

- Ciprofloxacin 500 mg orally two times per day for three days (not recommended for children or adolescents, nor during pregnancy or if breastfeeding).
- Erythromycin orally 1 g stat (immediately).
- Erythromycin 500 mg four times per day for seven days.

All sexual partners should also be treated, regardless of whether or not symptoms are present.

13.2: Lymphogranuloma venereum

History

Lymphogranuloma venereum (or LGV) is a contagious sexually transmitted infection (STI) affecting the lymph nodes in the groin, caused by the bacterium *Chlamydia trachomatis* (Figs. 13.2.1 and 13.2.2). The disease was first described by Wallace in 1833,

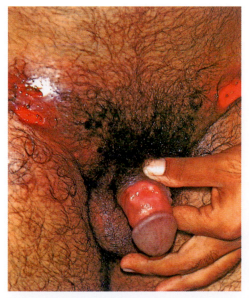

Figure 13.2.1: Lymphogranuloma venereum and syphilitic lesion. (Courtesy Dr N Khanna and Mehta Publishing House)

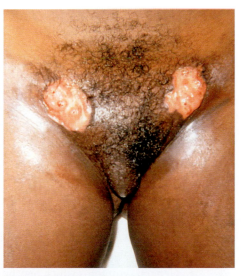

Figure 13.2.2: Lymphogranuloma venereum showing the typical groove sign due to enlargement of the femoral and inguinal lymph nodes. (Courtesy Dr N Khanna and Mehta Publishing House)

and subsequently fully characterised by NJ Durand, J Nicolas and M Favre in 1913 (hence its previous name of Durand–Nicolas–Favre disease). Lymphogranuloma venereum is found throughout the world but is particularly common in tropical and subtropical areas.

Causative organism

Lymphogranuloma venereum is caused by three strains of the bacterium *Chlamydia trachomatis*: L1, L2, and L3 (these strains are called serotypes and differ in their cell surface antigens).

Incubation period

This is of short duration, possibly 3 to 30 days.

Symptoms

There are three stages in the development of lymphogranuloma venereum:

- primary – initial lesion.
- secondary – multiple lesions with lymphadenopathy (also called bubo).
- tertiary – genito–anal–rectal syndrome.

Primary stage

- Papule or pustule at the site of inoculation (usually the genitals, but rarely in the mouth or other extragenital site), which becomes ulcerated and heals quickly.
- Multiple ulcers may appear on the prepuce, glans or scrotum in males or in the vaginal area, fourchette and vulva in females.

Secondary stage

This stage begins two to six weeks after appearance of the primary lesion. Symptoms are listed below.

- Inguinal lymphadenopathy – swollen lymph nodes in the groin are painful and often merge to form buboes.
- In females and homosexual males, perirectal nodes may be involved causing back pain.
- Suppurative granulomatous lymphadenitis may occur with nodes merging to form stellate abscesses.
- General symptoms which may be present:
  - fever (pyrexia).
  - headache.
  - arthralgia (joint pain).

Tertiary stage

This is the late manifestation of the disease which occurs several years after inoculation in the minority of patients who don't recover at the secondary stage. The tertiary stage is characterised by the following symptoms:

- proctitis – inflammation of the rectum lining with anal pruritus and rectal discharge.
- rectal bleeding or ulceration.
- genito–anal–rectal syndrome – rectal stricture.

Diagnosis

- Clinical presentation.
- Culture of swab from lesion – to identify *Chlamydia trachomatis*.
- PCR – to identify DNA specific to *Chlamydia trachomatis*.

Complications

- Lymphoedema – swelling or elephantiasis of the genitals (penis or vulva).
- Fistula – a connection from the rectum to the skin surface, often the result of a ruptured anal abscess.
- Rectal stricture.

Treatment

- Doxycycline 100 mg orally two times per day for three weeks.
- Erythromycin 500 mg four times per day for four weeks.

Treatment of complications

- Rectal stricture – may require surgery to drain pus and expand rectum.
- Fistula – surgery needed to correct.

All sexual partners should also be treated, regardless of whether symptoms are present.

13.3: Granuloma inguinale

History

Granuloma inguinale – also called ulcerative granuloma or Donovanosis – is a chronic sexually transmitted infection (STI) which mainly affects the skin of the genitalia. It was first reported in 1882 by K McLeod, a surgeon working in Calcutta, India, and further defined in 1905 by C Donovan who identified the presence of characteristic encapsulated rod-shaped bacilli (the causative bacterial organism) in patients' tissue samples or ulcer smears. These became known as 'Donovan bodies', hence the alternative name for the disease. Granuloma inguinale is endemic in many developing countries in tropical and subtropical areas, and relatively rare in developed countries. Sexually active people aged 20–40 years are most frequently affected.

Causative organism

The causative organism of granuloma inguinale is a bacillus called *Calymmatobacterium granulomatis* (previously called *Donovania granulomatis* after Donovan bodies). This is a gram-negative rod-shaped bacillus, 1.5 μm to 2.5 μm in length, found within the cytoplasm of host macrophages (white blood cells), and morphologically similar to species of the genus *Klebsiella*.

Mode of transmission

- Sexual contact.
- Skin contact.

Incubation period

Uncertain but may be approximately 60 days on average (suggested range: one day to one year).

Symptoms

Sites of involvement

- Genital organs – penis and scrotum in males; vulva, vagina and perineum in females.
- Inner thighs.
- Face.
- Anus and buttocks – in those practising anal intercourse.

The lesions characteristic of granuloma inguinale are:

- Papular or nodular lesion – soft and often pruritic, at inoculation site; this spreads via autoinoculation causing multiple lesions (Figs. 13.3.1 and 13.3.2).
- Ulcerative granulomatous mass – these raised, painless, ulcers develop from the soft nodules, and are large, red, and 'beefy' in appearance (Fig. 13.3.3).
- Ulcerative granulomatous lesion in the groin (Fig. 13.3.4).

Secondary bacterial infection of the ulcerative lesions is common. Lesions do not heal easily and may result in scarring. Lymph nodes are not involved.

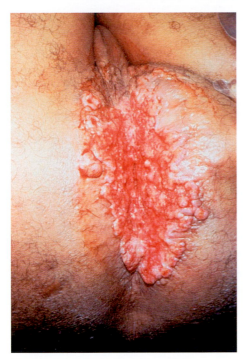

Figure 13.3.1: Granuloma inguinale. (Courtesy of CDC)

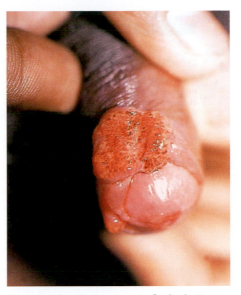

Figure 13.3.2: Donovanosis: fleshy lesions. (Courtesy Dr N Khanna and Mehta Publishing House)

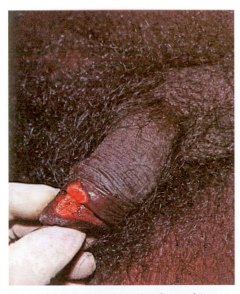

Figure 13.3.3: Donovanosis: clean, shiny, beefy red lesions with pearly border. (Courtesy Dr N Khanna and Mehta Publishing House)

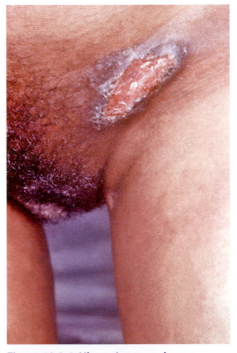

Figure 13.3.4: Ulcerative granulomatous lesion in the groin. (Courtesy of CDC)

Diagnosis

- Microscopic examination of lesion smear – Giemsa or Wright's stain to identify intracellular Donovan bodies characteristic of the disease.
- Biopsy from lesion – to identify Donovan bodies (usually used if unable to obtain fluid from dry lesions).
- PCR – to identify *C. granulomatis* DNA (test not commercially available).

Treatment

- Azithromycin 500 mg orally once daily for seven days.
- Erythromycin 500 mg four times per day for four weeks (in pregnancy).
- Ciprofloxacin 750 mg two times per day for three to five weeks.
- Doxycycline 100 mg orally two times per day for three weeks.

Sexual partners should also be treated regardless of whether symptoms are present. Follow-up of cases should be prolonged – up to six months may be required as lesions may be slow to heal.

Chapter 14: Non-venereal endemic treponematoses

14.1: Yaws

History

Yaws is a chronic infectious disease commonly found in tropical areas of Africa, South America, the Caribbean and Southeast Asia. The disease mostly occurs in children under the age of 15 years and has been known since at least 1679 in the Caribbean, where it was called 'yaya'.

Causative organism

Yaws is caused by the spirochaete bacterium *Treponema pallidum pertenue* (related to the bacterium that causes syphilis, but yaws is non-venereal). The bacterium was discovered by Aldo Castellani (1874–1971) in 1905.

Mode of transmission

As with the related conditions of pinta and bejel, yaws is transmitted by direct skin contact with an infected individual. There is some evidence of transmission from children to adults, but documented cases are relatively rare. Yaws is not classed as a sexually transmitted infection, despite *Treponema pallidum pertenue* being morphologically indistinguishable from *Treponema pallidum* – the causative agent of syphilis.

Incubation period

Yaws has an incubation period of three to five weeks.

Symptoms

There are two stages of yaws: early and late.

Early yaws

This is characterised by the primary and secondary stages of the disease:

- Primary: following infection, a papular lesion develops at the site of pathogen entry, which then ulcerates. This initial lesion is generally painless.
- Secondary: after three to six weeks of the primary skin lesion developing, systemic spread of the bacteria causes the appearance of multiple papillomatous skin lesions over the body. If lesions develop on the soles of the feet, they tend to have hard edges and are called 'crab-yaws'. Other signs of early yaws are characteristic bony lesions which may occur on the joints or the face (called gangosa). Mucous membranes may also be affected. The primary and secondary lesions of yaws are highly contagious.

Late yaws

In the late stage of yaws (also referred to as 'tertiary'), noticeable lesions are:

- plaque-like lesions.
- nodular scarring.
- ulcerative scarring.
- palmoplantar lesions.
- bone involvement (gangosa).

Late yaws is non-contagious and can occur after a long latency period, during which the disease may be asymptomatic. Cardiovascular and neurological involvement does not occur.

Diagnosis

- Clinical grounds – identification of *T. pallidum pertenue* from lesions.
- Non-treponemal serological tests, as for syphilis.
- Regional lymphadenopathy serology becomes positive during the first few weeks of infection.

Treatment

A single dose of benzathine penicillin 1.2 million units (MU) should be administered. For children less than 10 years old, the dose should be halved to 0.6 MU. If the patient is allergic to penicillin, the treatments of choice are erythromycin or tetracycline.

14.2: Pinta

History

Pinta is an ancient disease which has been recognised from the 16th century. In 1938, the disease was differentiated from syphilis and yaws by the identification of a separate causative spirochaete bacterium: *Treponema pallidum carateum*, although it is indistinguishable morphologically from *T. pallidum* and *T. pallidum pertenue* (the agents of syphilis and yaws, respectively). Pinta is an infectious disease, commonly affecting people in the age group 10 to 20 years in central and northern America.

Mode of transmission

Direct skin contact from person to person.

Incubation period

This is from two to three weeks.

Symptoms

As with other treponematoses, there are two stages: early and late.

Early pinta

This is characterised by the primary and secondary stages of the disease. An initial skin lesion is commonly present in the primary stage – seen as a papule on an exposed body part such as the foot, leg, forearm or hand, with multiple lesions characteristic of the secondary stage. There may also be regional lymphadenopathy.

Late pinta

This stage consists of a latent phase and a tertiary stage. The characteristic lesions are atrophic lesions similar to yaws, with changes to the skin pigment often present. Cardiovascular and neurological involvement does not occur.

Diagnosis

- Clinical grounds – identification of *T. pallidum carateum* from lesions.
- Non-treponemal serological tests, as for syphilis.

Treatment

A single dose of benzathine penicillin 1.2 million units (MU) should be administered. If the patient is allergic to penicillin, the treatments of choice are erythromycin or tetracycline.

14.3: Bejel

History

Bejel, or endemic syphilis, is a non-venereal contagious disease closely related to yaws and pinta. It was first fully described by EH Hudson in 1928, and is usually reported from the Middle East and Africa.

Causative organism

Bejel is caused by the spirochaete bacterium *Treponema pallidum endemicum*, which is indistinguishable from the *Treponema* species responsible for yaws, pinta (other non-venereal treponematoses) and syphilis.

Incubation period

This is from 10 to 90 days.

Mode of transmission

Close physical contact with an infected person, including sharing eating utensils.

Symptoms

- Skin rash at the inoculation site, spreading to other parts of the body.
- Primary lesions – usually painless – may present on the skin or in the oral cavity.
- Bony deformity – osteoperiostitis – typically in the leg bones (secondary stage).
- Ophthalmitis.
- Gummatous lesions – these cause deformity of bone and cartilage, typically of the nose (tertiary stage).

Diagnosis

- Clinical grounds – identification of *T. pallidum endemicum* from lesions.
- Serological tests, as for syphilis.

Treatment

A single dose of benzathine penicillin 1.2 million units (MU) should be administered. If the patient is allergic to penicillin, the treatments of choice are erythromycin or tetracycline.

Chapter 15: Urinary tract infection

Aetiology

Urinary tract infection (UTI) is a bacterial infection of either the upper (kidneys and ureters) or lower (bladder and urethra) urinary tract. Infections of the bladder and urethra cause cystitis and urethritis, respectively. The bacteria may enter the urethral opening following sexual intercourse, or less frequently the kidneys may be infected first, from blood-borne bacteria. UTI is very common and primarily affects females, but males may also be affected.

Causative organisms

Most UTIs are caused by bacteria that live in the alimentary canal and are transferred from the anus to the urethra during sexual intercourse or through poor personal hygiene. The causative bacterial species are:

- *Escherichia coli* (*E. coli*) – responsible for most UTI cases.
- *Staphylococcus saprophyticus* – responsible for up to 15% of cases.
- *Proteus mirabilis*, klebsiella and enterococci – gut flora rarely responsible for UTI.

Symptoms

Symptoms may be different for lower and upper UTIs.

Lower UTI

- Dysuria – pain or discomfort when passing urine.
- Cloudy urine.
- Frequent urge to pass urine.
- Haematuria – blood in urine.
- Lower abdominal tenderness or pain.
- Back pain.

Upper UTI

- Fever – lasting for at least two days.
- Shivering.

- Back pain – in the kidney area.
- Nausea.
- Vomiting.
- Diarrhoea.
- Symptoms of lower UTI may also be present.

Some people have bacteria present in their urine but have no other symptoms (asymptomatic bacteriuria). If left untreated, kidney infection (pyelonephritis) may develop in some cases.

Diagnosis

- Clinical presentation.
- Urine test – to identify causative bacteria.

Most cases do not require further diagnostic tests. If there is excessive blood in the urine, the following tests may be carried out to rule out more serious conditions or complications:

- ultrasound – this imaging technique can identify obstructions and causes of abnormal bladder emptying.
- intravenous urogram (IVU) – a dye is injected into the bloodstream so that the blood flow around the urinary tract can be viewed on X-ray.
- cystoscopy – the inside of the bladder is viewed with an instrument similar to an endoscope.

Complications

- Recurrent or persistent UTI – also called interstitial cystitis; small ulcers and haemorrhages may be present in the bladder.
- Pyelonephritis (kidney infection) – potentially serious condition that may result if UTI is left untreated; may lead to sepsis.
- Pregnancy – pregnant females are more likely to develop kidney infections from a UTI.

Treatment

Lower UTI

- Trimethoprim 200 mg orally two times per day for three days.
- Paracetamol or NSAIDs can be taken to relieve pain and discomfort.

Pregnant women and complicated cases should be prescribed a longer course of trimethoprim – at least seven days at the above dose.

Upper UTI

- Ciprofloxacin 500 mg orally two times per day for seven days.
- Paracetamol (but not NSAIDs) can be taken to relieve pain and discomfort.

Ciprofloxacin is not recommended in pregnancy: pregnant females should be prescribed cephalexin 250 mg to 1000 mg orally four times per day for 7 to 14 days. Hospital admission may be required for pregnant females, the elderly, or those with severe symptoms, diabetes or renal impairment.

Chapter 16: Genital herpes

Aetiology

Genital herpes is a chronic viral infection caused by the herpes simplex virus type 1 (HSV-1) or type 2 (HSV-2). The infection affects the genitalia, the anal area and occasionally the face of males and females. HSV-1 is the most common cause of genital herpes, although HSV-2 tends to recur more frequently than HSV-1. Genital herpes is a sexually transmitted infection with lesional contact being the primary route of transmission. Even if lesions are not visible, transmission may still occur during sexual contact from subclinical viral shedding.

After infection, the virus often lies dormant in the local sensory ganglion without symptoms. At intervals, the virus reactivates and becomes symptomatic, and recurrence is common.

Symptoms

HSV-1 and HSV-2 (Fig.16.1) produce the same symptoms.

- Lesions on the genitals, anus, or thighs – these are papular initially and then become vesicular and ulcerous (Figs. 16.2 to 16.9).

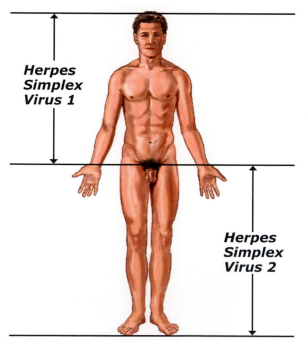

Figure 16.1: Herpes viruses.

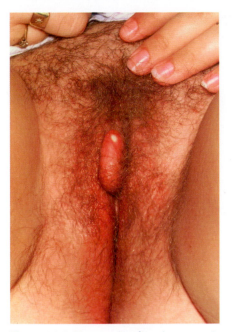

Figure 16.2: Herpes simplex virus type 1: on vulval area in a virgin girl.

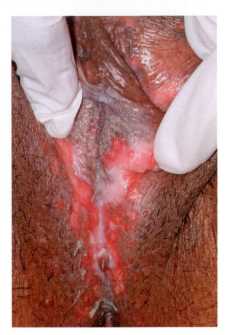

Figure 16.3: Genital herpes.

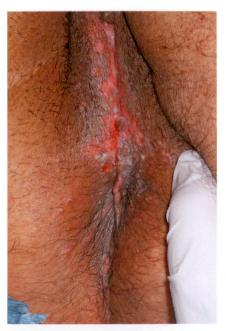

Figure 16.4: Genital herpes.

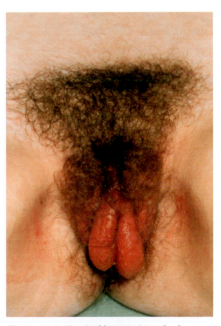

Figure 16.5: Genital herpes in vulval area.

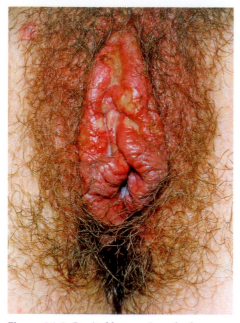

Figure 16.6: Genital herpes in vulval area.

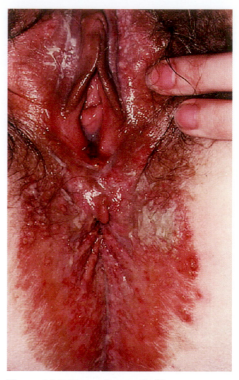

Figure 16.7: Extensive genital herpes.

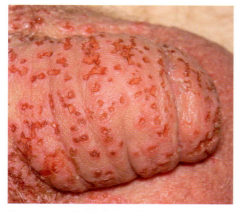

Figure 16.8: Herpes simplex virus type 2: herpes genitalis.

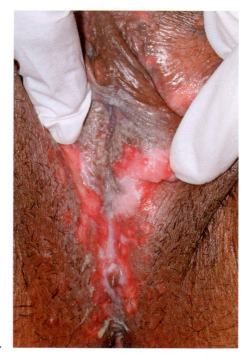

Figure 16.9: Adhesions due to herpes genitalis.

- Lesions on the cervix in females (Figs. 16.10 and 16.11).
- Vaginal discharge.
- Dysuria – pain when passing urine.
- Local adenitis – inflammation of lymph nodes.
- Fever.
- General malaise.
- Oral lesions on palatal area and tongue (Figs. 16.12 and 16.13).

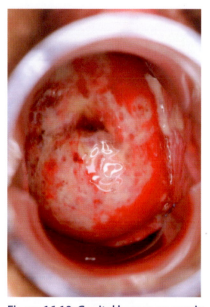

Figure 16.10: Genital herpes on cervix.

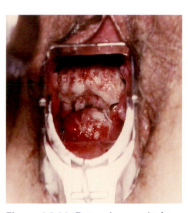

Figure 16.11: Extensive genital herpes on cervix.

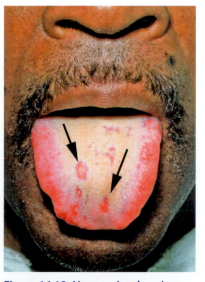

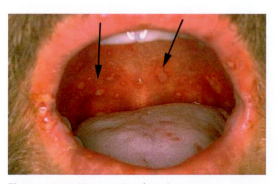

Figure 16.12: Herpes simplex virus type 1: on palatal area.

Figure 16.13: Herpes simplex virus type 1: on tongue.

- Cold sore (Figs. 16.14 and 16.15).
- Extensive herpetic lesions in groin area (Fig. 16.16).
- Typical herpetic vesicles (Fig. 16.17).

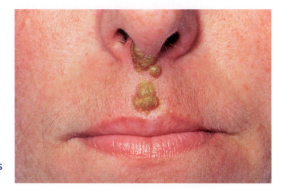

Figure 16.14: Herpes simplex virus type 1: cold sore on upper lip.

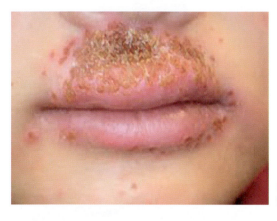

Figure 16.15: Herpes simplex virus type 1: cold sore on upper lip.

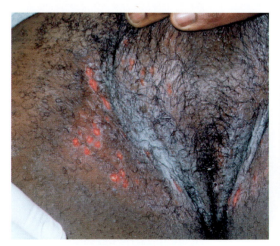

Figure 16.16: Genital herpes in groin.

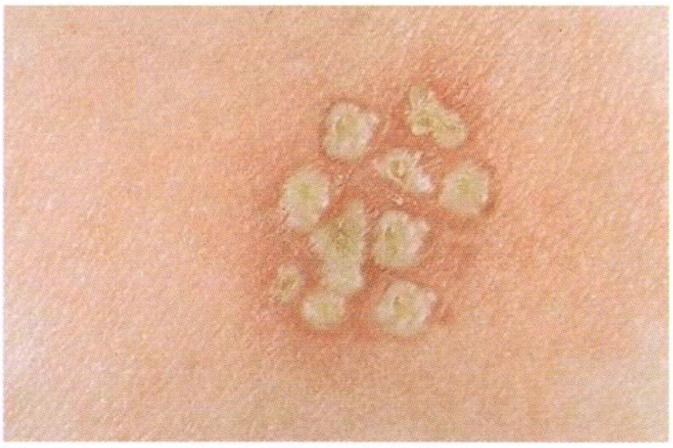

Figure 16.17: Herpes vesicles.

Diagnosis

- Clinical presentation.
- Laboratory methods
  - PCR of lesion swab – very specific test which can identify HSV DNA and type.
  - Virus culture from lesion swab – very specific test that confirms HSV and type (1 or 2), and allows testing of antiviral medication sensitivity.
  - Enzyme immunoassay of lesion swab – detects antigens specific to HSV (but cannot differentiate types); not as sensitive as the above methods.
  - Immunofluorescence of smear – as for EIA.
- Serological assays – these detect specific antibodies to HSV and are indicated for patients with a first episode of HSV, those with recurrent or atypical genital disease, and sexual partners.
  - Western blot – gold standard for diagnosis but not commercially available.
  - Commercial HSV detection kits (e.g. Focus HerpeSelect ELISA; HerpeSelect immunoblot; Kalon HSV-2) are highly specific and offer higher than 95% sensitivity.

Early infection may produce false negatives in serological tests. Repeat testing is recommended. HSV type can be diagnosed from IgG antibodies 2 to 12 weeks after the appearance of symptoms.

Complications

Possible complications which may require hospitalisation include urinary retention, meningitis and severe malaise. Secondary infection of lesions may occur and adhesions may result if herpes genitalis is present (see Fig. 16.9, page 86).

Treatment

First episode genital herpes

Oral antiviral drugs should be administered within five days of the appearance of symptoms in one of the following regimens:

- aciclovir 200 mg five times per day for five days.
- aciclovir 400 mg three times per day for five days.
- famciclovir 250 mg three times per day for five days.
- valaciclovir 500 mg two times per day for five days.

Analgesics may also be taken for symptomatic pain relief. Counselling should be given to patients and sexual partners to reduce the chance of future HSV contact.

Recurrent genital herpes

Oral antiviral drugs can reduce the duration and severity of recurrent HSV episodes, particularly if administered within 24 hours of the appearance of symptoms using one of the following regimens:

- aciclovir 200 mg five times per day for five days.
- aciclovir 400 mg three times per day for three to five days.
- aciclovir 800 mg three times per day for two days.
- famciclovir 125 mg two times per day for five days.
- famciclovir 1 g two times per day for one day.
- valaciclovir 500 mg two times per day for three to five days.

Suppressive treatment for patients with at least six episodes of HSV per year may be necessary, as follows:

- aciclovir 400 mg two times per day for 6 to 12 months.
- valaciclovir 250 mg two times per day for 6 to 12 months.

Immunocompromised and HIV-positive patients

The following regimens can be used but the duration of antiviral therapy may need to be extended until the lesions have recovered:

- aciclovir 200–400 mg five times per day for 5 to 10 days.
- aciclovir 400–800 mg three times per day for 5 to 10 days.
- famciclovir 250–500 mg three times per day for 5 to 10 days.
- valaciclovir 500–1000 mg two times per day for 5 to 10 days.

Suppressive treatment for patients with at least six episodes of HSV per year:

- aciclovir 400–800 mg two times per day for 6 to 12 months.
- valaciclovir 500–1000 mg two times per day for 6 to 12 months.
- alternative if the above regimens fail: famciclovir 500 mg two times per day for 6 to 12 months.

Pregnancy

HSV infection in the first and second trimester should be treated with oral or intravenous aciclovir at standard doses. For women in the third trimester, treatment should be aciclovir 400 mg three times per day from week 36 of the pregnancy to prevent HSV lesions at the due date.

If symptoms are present during the last six weeks of the pregnancy, caesarean section should be considered due to risk of passing the virus to the baby during labour. Babies born to mothers with genital HSV lesions should be tested for HSV and intravenous aciclovir therapy initiated as required.

Chapter 17: Human papillomavirus

Aetiology

The human papillomavirus is a virus with many different strains (approximately 150), some of which are sexually transmitted and cause either genital warts or dysplasia. Genital warts are small benign growths (papillomas) on the skin in the genital area which, although unsightly, are not a serious medical problem. Dysplasia is abnormal cells of the cervix in females, which may be a precursor to cervical cancer.

HPV types are classified as low-risk (those that don't cause cancer) and high-risk (those that can lead to cancers):

- Low risk types
  - HPV-6, HPV-11, HPV-42, HPV-43, HPV-44, HPV-54, HPV-61, HPV-70, HPV-72, HPV-81.
- High-risk types
  - HPV-16, HPV-18, HPV-31, HPV-33, HPV-35, HPV-39, HPV-45, HPV-51, HPV-52, HPV-56, HPV-58, HPV-59, HPV-68, HPV-73, HPV-82.

Genital warts

Genital warts are caused by low-risk HPV types, the majority being due to HPV-6 and HPV-11, with the remainder being caused by HPV-42, HPV-43 and HPV-44. Genital warts are benign tumours but will continue to grow if not treated and are highly contagious.

Sites of involvement

Genital warts – also referred to as anogenital warts or condylomata acuminata – occur in males and females at any of the following sites:

- Males.
  - penis shaft.
  - glans penis.
  - scrotum.
- Females
  - vagina – around or inside.
  - vulva.
  - cervix.

- Males and females.
  - urethra.
  - inner thigh.
  - anus – around or inside.
  - mouth or throat – in those practising oral sex with an infected individual.

Mode of transmission

- Sexual contact.
- Intimate physical contact.
- Anal sex.
- Oral sex.

Incubation period

Genital warts usually appear one to six months after exposure, but it may be up to several years. In some cases individuals may be carriers of HPV and never develop genital warts.

Types of wart

- Follicular – warts that grow from a hair follicle; may occur in the genital area or other places on the body (Fig. 17.1).

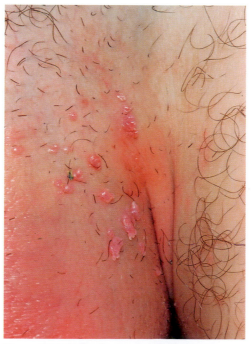

Figure 17.1: Follicular warts in vulval area.

- Filiform – longer, thinner, warts which can occur on the genitals or other areas such as eyelids.
- Keratinised – firm warts found on more-keratinised skin, such as the penis shaft.
- Soft – these warts occur on softer, non-keratinised skin such as the vulva, anus and foreskin.
- Hyperkeratotic – warts in which the surrounding skin is thickened and hard (Fig. 17.2).
- Cauliflower – clusters of warts in a round, rough, formation with the appearance of a cauliflower (Fig. 17.3).
- Seborrhoeic – usually highly pigmented or black warts with a rough, raised, surface and defined border (Figs. 17.4, 17.5 and 17.6).

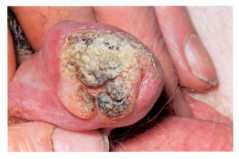

Figure 17.2: Hyperkeratotic warts.

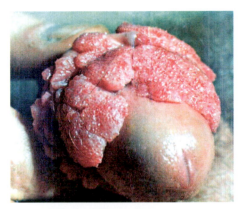

Figure 17.3: Cauliflower warts.

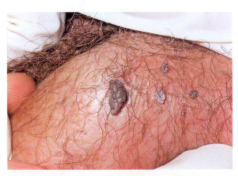

Figure 17.4: Seborrhoeic warts.

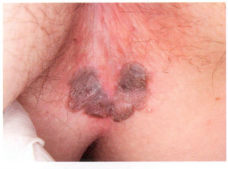

Figure 17.5: Seborrhoeic warts.

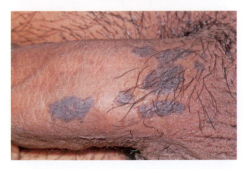

Figure 17.6: Seborrhoeic warts on the shaft of the penis.

Symptoms

- Itching.
- Irritation or redness in the genital area.
- New growths on the skin in the genital area.
- Pain during intercourse – especially if penile or vaginal warts are present.
- Bleeding during intercourse.
- Dysuria (difficulty passing urine) – warts in the urethra.
- Pain in the mouth or difficulty swallowing – warts in the mouth, on the tongue or lip.

Sites for warts

- Meatal (Fig. 17.7).
- Vulval (Figs. 17.8, 17.9 and 17.10).
- Preputial (Fig. 17.11).
- Extensive soft warts on the prepuce and glans penis (Fig. 17.12).
- Warts on the tongue (Figs. 17.13 and 17.14, page 96).
- Warts on the lip (Fig. 17.15, page 96).
- Wart on the nipple (Fig. 17.16, page 96).

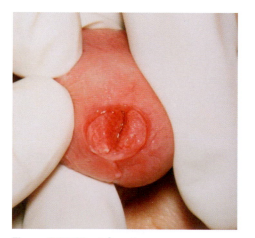

Figure 17.7: Meatal warts.

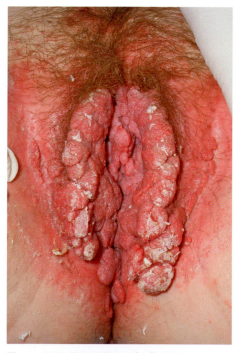

Figure 17.8: Extensive vulval warts.

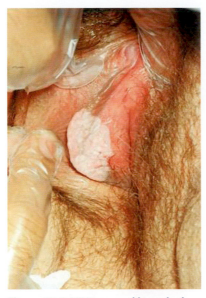

Figure 17.9: VIN2 caused by vulval wart.

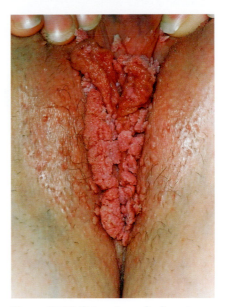

Figure 17.10: Extensive vulval warts.

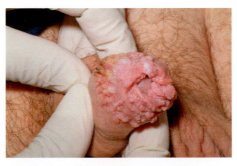

Figure 17.11: Preputial warts.

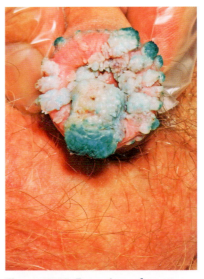

Figure 17.12: Extensive soft warts on penis.

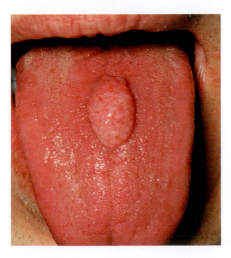

Figure 17.13: Warts on the tongue.

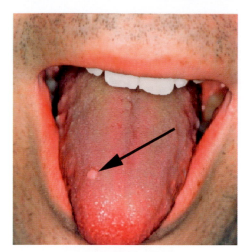

Figure 17.14: Warts on the tongue.

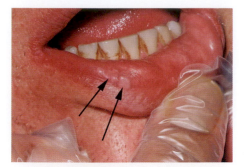

Figure 17.15: Warts on the lower lip.

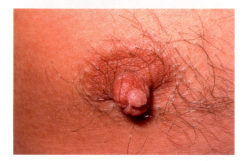

Figure 17.16: Wart on the nipple of a homosexual patient.

- Perianal warts (Figs. 17.17 and 17.18).
- Cervical warts (Fig. 17.19).
- Penile intraepithelial neoplasia (PIN-2) caused by penile warts (Fig. 17.20, page 98).
- Care should be taken to differentiate between warts and papillomatous lesions (Fig. 17.21, page 98) which look similar to warts but require different treatment.

Diagnosis

- Clinical presentation.
- Pap smear test (Papanicolaou or cervical smear test) – for females, to determine any changes to the cervix due to genital warts.

Complications

- Infection with high-risk HPV may lead to cervical, vaginal, anal or penile cancers.
- Pregnancy – vaginal warts may reduce the elasticity of the vaginal wall during childbirth.

Treatment

- Imiquimod cream 5%, applied to warts three times per week for 16 weeks – this strengthens the ability of the immune system to fight the HPV virus.

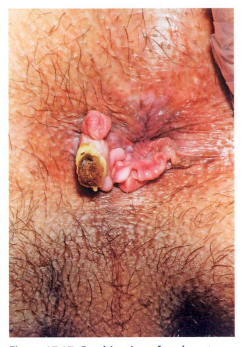

Figure 17.17: Combination of anal warts and haemorrhoids.

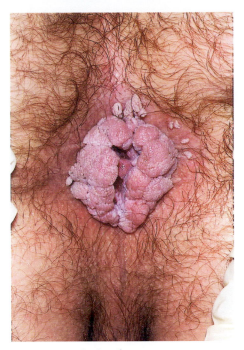

Figure 17.18: Perianal warts.

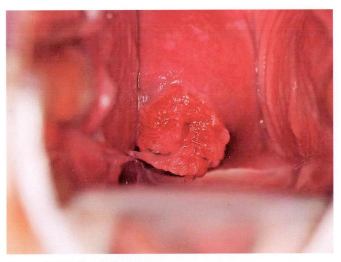

Figure 17.19: Cervical wart.

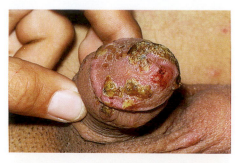
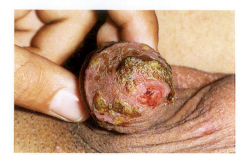
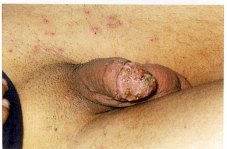

Figure 17.20: PIN-2 caused by penile warts.

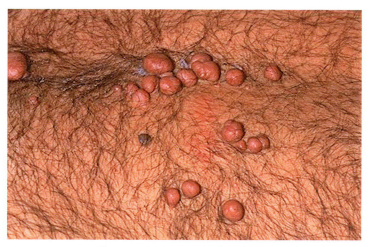

Figure 17.21: Papillomatous lesions which look similar to warts.

- Podophyllotoxin solution or cream 0.5%, applied two times per day for three days, followed by four days without treatment; repeated for four weeks.
- Podophyllin solution 10% to 25% – this treatment is administered in clinic as it is toxic and needs to be washed off within four hours.
- TCA (trichloroacetic acid) – this acid burns out the warts and is administered in clinic.

- Cryosurgery – this destroys the wart by freezing with liquid nitrogen.
- Electrocautery – an electrical current produces heat to burn off warts.
- Surgery – warts can be cut out under local anaesthetic.
- Laser treatment – only usually used for large and treatment-resistant warts.

Dysplasia

Dysplasia is caused by high-risk HPV types, mostly HPV-16 and HPV-18, with the remainder being caused by HPV-31, HPV-33, HPV-35, HPV-39, HPV-45, HPV-51, HPV-52, HPV-56 and HPV-58. Dysplasia is a precancerous state of the cervix, but it is very treatable and only 2% of cases actually develop into cancer.

Grading of dysplasia

The severity of cervical dysplasia may range from very mild to severe. The grading scale used to assess severity is the cervical intraepithelial neoplasia CIN-1, 2 or 3 system, where the grading is:

- CIN-1 – mild dysplasia, affecting only the basal third of the cervical lining thickness, including the epithelium.
- CIN-2 – moderate dysplasia, with abnormalities affecting the basal two-thirds of the cervical lining thickness.
- CIN-3 – severe dysplasia, with precancerous changes to cells over more than two-thirds of the cervical lining thickness, including full-thickness lesions.

High-risk HPV types can also cause precancerous changes to cells on the vulva (vulval intraepithelial neoplasia or VIN), the perianal and anal area (perianal and anal intraepithelial neoplasia or PAIN), and the penis (penis intraepithelial neoplasia or PIN). As with CIN, these conditions are graded VIN-1, 2 or 3, PAIN-1, 2 or 3, and PIN-1, 2 or 3, respectively.

Symptoms

Many cases of dysplasia caused by HPV are asymptomatic and are only detected from routine Pap smear tests. The following symptoms may occur:

- bloody discharge from the vagina – due to bleeding from the cervix.
- irritation.
- pain – at the vulva, cervix, perianal area or penis.
- flaking of the skin or tissue.

Diagnosis

- Clinical presentation.
- Pap smear test – this will identify the abnormal cells on the cervix.

- Colposcopy – a binocular microscope is used to examine the walls of the vagina and the cervix to identify abnormalities following a Pap smear.
- Biopsy – tissue sample taken for analysis following positive result from colposcopy.
- HPV DNA test – cells from the cervix (or from the vulva, perianal/anal area, or penis for cases of VIN, PAIN or PIN) can be tested to identify high-risk HPV strains from viral DNA.
- Women over 30 years of age may have a routine HPV DNA test, regardless of Pap test results.

Complications

Cancer may result if cervical, vulval, perianal/anal or penile intraepithelial neoplasia goes untreated.

Treatment

CIN-1

Usually resolves spontaneously so no treatment is necessary. Regular follow-up is required to ensure it doesn't progress to CIN-2. Cases of CIN-2 and CIN-3 may be treated as follows:

CIN-2

- Carbon dioxide laser photoablation – this destroys the abnormal cells; administered under local anaesthetic.
- Cryosurgery – this destroys the abnormal cells by freezing them with liquid nitrogen; only used for small areas of disease.

CIN-3

- Loop electrosurgical excision (LEEP) – a radiofrequency current is used to remove abnormal tissue, which can then be analysed for possible cancer.
- Hysterectomy – surgical removal of the uterus, including the cervix; used for severe cases of dysplasia and for cervical cancer.

The above treatments also apply to cases of VIN, PAIN and PIN. In addition, these high-risk HPV infections may be treated similarly to genital warts using the following:

- Imiquimod cream 5% – applied to the affected area three times per week for 16 weeks.
- 5-fluorouracil cream 5% – applied to the affected area two times per day until abnormal tissue is destroyed.
- Podophyllotoxin solution or cream 0.5%, applied two times per day for three days, followed by four days without treatment; repeated for four weeks.

- Podophyllin solution 10% to 25% – administered in clinic due to its toxicity and needs to be washed off within four hours.
- TCA (trichloroacetic acid) – this acid treatment is administered in clinic.
- Cryosurgery – liquid nitrogen kills the abnormal cells.
- Electrocautery – electrically-induced heat burns off the affected tissue.
- Laser treatment – burns off the affected tissue.

Risk factors

- Multiple sexual partners – more chances of exposure to HPV.
- Smoking – chemicals in cigarette smoke are linked with dysplasia.
- Other sexually transmitted infections – HIV in particular may predispose females to high-risk HPV infection and dysplasia.
- Low levels of folic acid – possibly due to use of oral contraceptives.

Vaccination for HPV

Risk of cervical cancer can be reduced by vaccination against HPV. The two vaccines available are:

- Cervarix – this protects against HPV types 16 and 18, which cause approximately 75% of all cases of cervical cancer. Protection is long-term, and all girls aged 13 years and over are offered this vaccine by the United Kingdom National Health Service.
- Gardasil – provides protection against HPV types 6 and 11 (which cause 90% of cases of genital warts) and HPV types 16 and 18 (which cause approximately 75% of all cases of cervical cancer).
- The vaccination schedule should include injections at month 0, month 2 and month 6.

Chapter 18: Molluscum contagiosum

History

Molluscum contagiosum is a contagious viral disease of the skin characterised by pinhead or pea-sized papules, which may be whitish or pink in colour. The disease was first described by Bateman in 1817 but the viral cause was not identified until 1905, by Juliusberg. It is prevalent throughout the world and children are most often affected but it also occurs in adults, in whom it is considered a sexually transmitted infection.

Causative organism

The disease is caused by a member of the poxvirus family. There are four viral subtypes of the molluscum contagiosum virus (MCV), MCV 1, 2, 3 and 4, and all produce the same types of symptoms.

Mode of transmission

- Direct skin contact.
- Sharing towels, bed sheets or clothes with an infected individual.
- Sexual contact.

Incubation period

Generally two to seven weeks from initial exposure, but may be up to six months.

Symptoms

Molluscum contagiosum affects the skin (and occasionally mucous membranes) on all parts of the body except the palms and the soles. When sexually transmitted, lesions may appear in the genital area in both males and females, including the shaft of the penis, scrotal area, vulva and groin. Lesions may be as follows:

- Papular lesions (3 mm to 9 mm in diameter), firm and hemispherical (Figs. 18.1 and 18.2).
- Pearly or flesh-coloured umbilicated (central depression) lesions; these may enlarge to become nodules.
- Lesions may have a white, milky or waxy core.

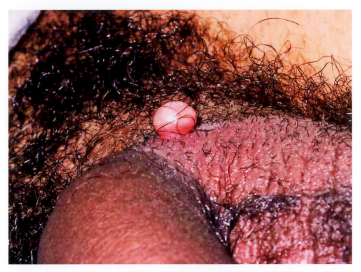

Figure 18.1: Solitary molluscum contagiosum.

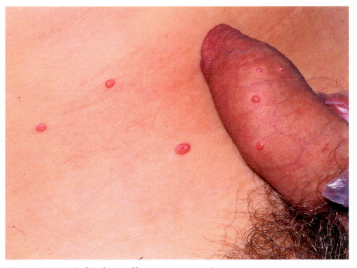

Figure 18.2: Multiple molluscum contagiosum.

- Lesions are painless and non-itchy unless they become inflamed.
- An impaired immune system (e.g. due to AIDS) can aid the development of more numerous and larger lesions.

Diagnosis

- Clinical presentation of lesions.
- Biopsy of lesion core – to identify characteristic molluscum inclusion bodies.

Complications

- Secondary infection of lesions.
- Persistent spread of lesions due to autoinoculation.
- Recurrence of lesions.

Treatment

Molluscum contagiosum is usually self-limiting and symptoms may disappear in several months to about three years. Large, troublesome or persistent lesions may be treated as follows:

- Cryotherapy (liquid nitrogen) – to freeze and remove lesions.
- Trichloroacetic acid.
- Curettage – scraping lesions off the skin with a metal instrument.
- Diathermy – electrically produced heat treatment.
- Laser treatment.
- Imiquimod – topical immune-activating cream.

Patients should be followed up regularly as repeat treatment every two or three weeks may be necessary to completely remove the disease. Where appropriate, sexual partners should also be screened and treated.

Chapter 19: Sexually acquired viral hepatitis B and C

Aetiology

Viral hepatitis is inflammation of the liver caused by one of several strains of the hepatitis virus, which include A, B, C, D, E and G. The infection may be acute or chronic and is transmitted via blood and bodily fluids such as saliva and semen. Of the hepatitis strains, hepatitis B is well known to be transmitted by sexual contact, and recent evidence indicates that hepatitis C is also a sexually transmitted infection.

Hepatitis B

Hepatitis B is one of the most frequent and widespread contagious diseases in the world, with prevalence being highest in African, Asian and South American countries. Sexual contact is a major route of transmission, in both heterosexual and homosexual relationships. Infected mothers may also pass the infection to their newborn children during childbirth.

Incubation period

Generally 40 to 90 days after infection, but can be up to six months.

Symptoms

Hepatitis B may be asymptomatic, but some or all of the following symptoms may be present:

- fatigue.
- loss of appetite – may lead to weight loss.
- nausea – with or without vomiting.
- abdominal pain.
- jaundice – yellowing of the skin and the whites of the eyes (Fig. 19.1, next page).
- dark urine.
- grey or white stools.
- joint pain.

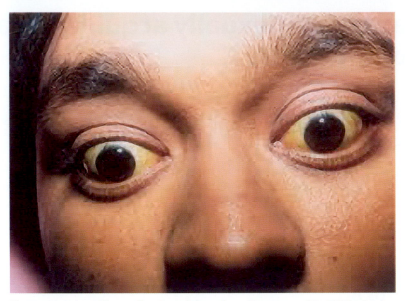

Figure 19.1: Jaundice: yellowing of the sclera. (Courtesy of Dr DK Kochar)

Diagnosis

Following clinical presentation of any of the above symptoms, diagnosis of hepatitis B can be confirmed by tests for specific markers of *Hepatitis B virus* and tests of liver function.

- Hepatitis B surface antigen (HBsAg): a specific serological marker on the surface of the *Hepatitis B virus*. It is present in high levels in serum during acute and chronic hepatitis B, and indicates that the person is infectious. As part of the normal immune response to the infection, the body produces antibodies to HBsAg.

- Hepatitis B surface antibody (anti-HBs): the presence of anti-HBs usually indicates recovery and immunity from hepatitis B infection. Anti-HBs is also found in people who have been successfully vaccinated against hepatitis B.

- Total hepatitis B core antibody (anti-HBc): this is an antibody to the virus core antigen, which appears at the onset of symptoms in acute hepatitis B and persists for life. The presence of anti-HBc indicates previous or ongoing infection with the *Hepatitis B virus* in an undefined time frame.

- IgM antibody to hepatitis B core antigen (IgM anti-HBc): this antibody appears during acute or recent hepatitis B infection and is present for about six months, during which time it may be the largest constituent of the total hepatitis B core antibody (anti-HBc) count.

- Liver function tests – If hepatitis B has been confirmed, blood samples should be tested to identify liver damage caused by the *Hepatitis B virus*.
  - Alanine aminotransferase (ALT) – levels of this liver enzyme are raised in hepatitis B.

- Aspartate aminotransferase (AST) – levels of this liver enzyme are raised in hepatitis B, but not as specific as ALT.
- Alkaline phosphatase (ALP) – this enzyme is found in liver cells associated with bile ducts; levels are raised in hepatitis B.
- Albumin – the primary protein made by the liver; levels of albumin in the blood may be reduced.
- Total protein (including albumin) – may be reduced.
- Bilirubin – this is a chemical pigment present in blood, resulting from the breakdown of haemoglobin. In hepatitis B, high levels of direct (conjugated) bilirubin in the blood produce the yellow skin colour of jaundice, indicating a reduced ability of the liver to remove it.

- False positives
  - AST levels can be raised when heart or skeletal muscle is damaged; the ALT test is more specific to hepatitis.
  - ALP levels may be raised in some bone diseases.
  - Bilirubin (conjugated) levels can be raised when the bile duct is blocked due to a gallstone or a pancreatic tumour. Alcoholism may also cause liver damage leading to raised bilirubin levels.

Complications

- Cirrhosis of the liver – in chronic infections (longer than six months duration), which may lead to liver cancer.
- Hepatitis B can be passed from an infected mother to her newborn baby during childbirth.
- Fulminant hepatitis – a severe form of acute hepatitis causing total liver failure and often hepatic encephalopathy, coma, kidney failure and death.

Treatment

Acute hepatitis B usually resolves spontaneously, so no treatment is required. If a patient has chronic, active hepatitis B with replicating virus, the following treatments should be administered:

- interferon alpha-2b (an immune modulator which helps the patient's immune system fight the infection) 3 million units (MU) – administered intramuscular three times per week
- alternatively: pegylated interferon alpha-2b (a long-acting version) 180 µg – administered intramuscular once weekly
- antiviral drugs (these stop the virus replicating):
  - entecavir 0.5 mg orally once daily, available as a tablet or liquid suspension (if previously resistant to lamivudine, the dose should be 1 g once daily).
  - adefovir dipivoxil 10 mg orally once daily (not recommended for children under 12 years of age).

- telbivudine 600 mg orally once daily, available as a tablet or liquid suspension (not recommended for children under 16 years of age).
- tenofovir disoproxil fumarate 300 mg orally once daily (not recommended for children or adolescents with hepatitis B).
- lamivudine 100 mg orally once daily in adults. For children two years of age and above, dose at 3 mg/kg bodyweight orally once daily, to a maximum of 100 mg per day.

Treatments for hepatitis B should be continued long term. Discontinuing treatment may lead to severe relapse of the disease. If this occurs, treatment should be resumed. Patients should be regularly monitored during and after treatment.

Screening and vaccination

Hepatitis B screening and vaccination is indicated in the following patient groups:

- people coming from areas where hepatitis B is endemic, such as China, parts of Asia and some African countries.
- homosexuals – particularly men who have sex with other men (MSM).
- healthcare professionals, including paramedics.
- sex industry workers.
- rape cases.
- human bite injuries (post-exposure prophylaxis – PEP).
- needle stick injuries (PEP).
- people who have had casual sex with a person who may be infected with HIV (PEP).
- all HIV cases.
- intravenous drug users.

The three patient groups in the above list indicated for post-exposure prophylaxis (PEP) should be screened (including testing for HBsAg) and vaccinated for hepatitis B within 72 hours of contact or injury. Routine blood tests (liver function tests, urea and electrolytes and full blood picture) should also be carried out on the first day, after seven days and after four weeks. In addition, tests for HIV and hepatitis C antibodies (HCA) are necessary.

There are three types of vaccination schedule.

- Standard:
  - same day.
  - after one month.
  - after six months.
- Accelerated:
  - same day.
  - after one month.
  - after two months.
  - after one year.

- Super accelerated:
  - same day.
  - after seven days.
  - after three weeks.
  - after one year.

Ideally, vaccination for hepatitis B should be started on the same day, on a 'super accelerated' schedule.

Eight weeks after finishing the full vaccination schedule, the patient should be tested for hepatitis B antibodies (HbsAb): if the result is less than 10, the full course of vaccination should be repeated or a booster vaccination administered. The hepatitis B vaccine is a preparation of hepatitis surface antigen protein (HbsAg), and is commercially available as Engerix-B 20 μg/mL, administered intramuscularly.

Where immunisation has been delayed beyond the recommended intervals, the vaccine course should be completed, but it is more likely that the child may become infected. In this instance, testing for HBsAg above the age of one year is particularly important.

Interrupted vaccine schedules

- When the hepatitis B vaccine schedule is interrupted, the vaccine series does not need to be restarted.
- If the series is interrupted after the first dose, the second dose should be administered as soon as possible, and the second and third doses should be separated by an interval of at least eight weeks.
- If only the third dose has been delayed, it should be administered as soon as possible.

Minimum dosing intervals and management of persons who were vaccinated incorrectly

- The third dose of vaccine must be administered at least eight weeks after the second dose and at least 16 weeks after the first dose; the minimum interval between the first and second doses is four weeks.
- Inadequate doses of hepatitis B vaccine or doses received after a shorter-than-recommended dosing interval should be re-administered, using the correct dosage or schedule.

Hepatitis C

Hepatitis C is widespread and highly prevalent with up to 5% of the population in developing countries carrying the disease. Areas particularly affected are China and Africa. As with hepatitis B, hepatitis C is transmitted via blood and bodily fluids, so can be transmitted during sexual contact. Co-infection with HIV increases the transmission rate.

Other routes of transmission include sharing of infected needles and receiving infected blood products.

Incubation period

Up to 150 days after infection in patients with acute hepatitis C, but most cases are asymptomatic with chronic hepatitis C developing up to 20 years after the initial infection.

Symptoms

Hepatitis C is initially asymptomatic in about 80% of cases, but some or all of the following symptoms may eventually be present during acute or chronic infections:

- fatigue.
- loss of appetite – may lead to weight loss.
- nausea – with or without vomiting.
- abdominal pain.
- jaundice (in acute infections) – yellowing of the skin and the whites of the eyes.
- dark urine.
- grey or white stools.
- flu-like symptoms.
- joint pain.

Diagnosis

Following clinical presentation of any of the above symptoms, diagnosis of hepatitis C can be confirmed by tests for specific markers of *Hepatitis C virus* and tests of liver function.

- Antibody test (anti-HCV) – the presence of antibodies to the virus indicates exposure to hepatitis C.
- Recombinant immunoblot assay (RIBA) test – used to confirm the presence of antibodies to hepatitis C.
- Polymerase chain reaction test – detects active viral RNA – genetic material specific to hepatitis C.
- Liver function tests – blood samples are tested to identify liver damage due to the *Hepatitis C virus*:
  - Alanine aminotransferase (ALT) – levels of this liver enzyme are raised in hepatitis C.
  - Aspartate aminotransferase (AST) – levels of this liver enzyme are raised in hepatitis C, but not as specific as ALT.
  - Alkaline phosphatase (ALP) – this enzyme is found in liver cells associated with bile ducts; levels are raised in hepatitis C.
  - Albumin – the primary protein made by the liver; levels of albumin in the blood may be reduced.

- Total protein (including albumin) – may be reduced.
- Bilirubin – this is a chemical pigment present in blood, resulting from the breakdown of haemoglobin. In hepatitis C, high levels of direct (conjugated) bilirubin in the blood produce the yellow skin colour of jaundice, indicating a reduced ability of the liver to remove it.
- False positives.
  - The antibody test and the RIBA test may give positive results even when a patient no longer has hepatitis C infection because antibodies to the virus can remain in the body for several years after recovery.
  - AST levels can be raised when heart or skeletal muscle is damaged; the ALT test is more specific to hepatitis.
  - ALP levels may be raised in some bone diseases.
  - Bilirubin (conjugated) levels can be raised when the bile duct is blocked due to a gallstone or a pancreatic tumour. Alcoholism may cause liver damage leading to raised bilirubin levels.

Complications

- Cirrhosis of the liver – in chronic infections (longer than six months duration), which may lead to liver cancer.
- Fulminant hepatitis – a severe form of acute hepatitis causing total liver failure and often hepatic encephalopathy, coma, kidney failure and death.

Treatment

Acute hepatitis C may resolve spontaneously, in which case no treatment is required. If a patient has symptomatic acute or chronic hepatitis C, the following treatments should be administered:

- interferon alpha-2b (an immune modulator which helps the patient's immune system fight the infection) 3 million units (MU) – administered intramuscular three times per week.
- alternatively: pegylated interferon alpha-2b (a long-acting version) 180 µg – administered intramuscular once weekly.
- ribavirin 1 g orally once daily in combination with interferon alpha-2b or pegylated interferon alpha-2b – it is not effective on its own. If the patient weighs more than 75 kg, the dose should be 1.2 g once daily.

Treatment for hepatitis C should be continued for 6 to 12 months. Patients should be regularly monitored during and after treatment and retreatment may be necessary.

Chapter 20: Scabies

History

According to the literature, Giovan Cosimo Bonomo in collaboration with Diacinto Cestoni discovered the scabies mite in 1687. They identified this arachnoid parasite (*Sarcoptes scabiei* var. hominis) (Fig. 20.1) – related to spiders and scorpions – as the cause of the disease. This parasite also causes mange in animals.

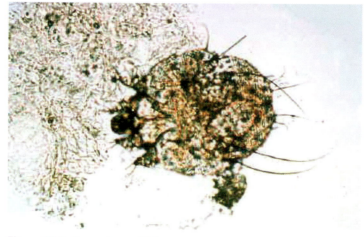

Figure 20.1: *Sarcoptes scabiei.*

Aetiology

The adult mite burrows into the stratum corneum of the skin (the upper layer of the epidermis), where the female lays eggs. The burrows may be 5 mm in length and visible to the naked eye (Neynaber and Wolff, 2008). After two to three days, eggs hatch into larvae which then excavate new burrows. Here, after about four days, the larvae hatch into nymphs, which then undergo two further moults before emerging as adult mites. The adult mite has four pairs of legs and a round body with no distinct head. The female mite is 0.4 mm in size, whereas the male is 0.25 mm. Newly matured female mites dig a short burrow in the skin and wait for a male to find them. Mating occurs and the cycle repeats. After copulation the male dies and the female lays three to four eggs in a shallow burrow every day. During an adult female's life cycle of one to two months, she may lay from 150 to 180 eggs. Scabies is classed as a sexually transmitted disease.

Incubation period

The incubation period is two to six weeks, occasionally less.

Mode of transmission

Close physical contact with a person with the infestation, crowded living conditions, poor personal hygiene; may be more prevalent in low socioeconomic groups.

Symptoms

- Intense itching.
- Generalised papular eruption.
- Nocturnal itching.
- Characteristic lesions formed by the burrows made by female mites.
- Parts of the body affected (Figs. 20.2 and 20.3).
    - interdigital clefts of the hands.
    - flexor surfaces of the wrist, elbow and axillary folds.
    - buttocks.

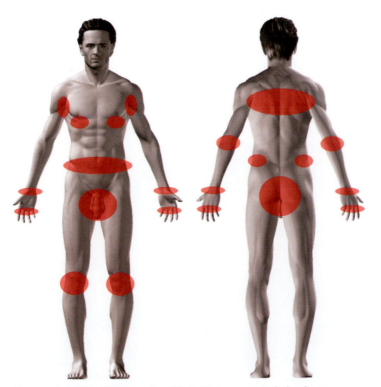

Figure 20.2: Distribution of scabietic lesions on male body areas.

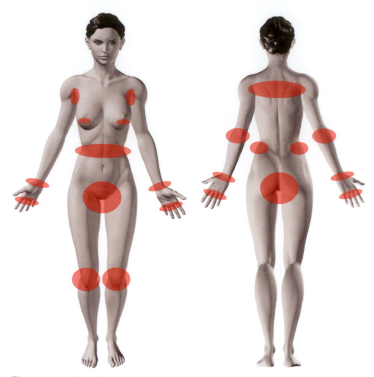

Figure 20.3: Distribution of scabietic lesions on female body areas.

– male genitalia (Figs. 20.4 to 20.7).
– female areola of the breast.
– in children, the palmar area, head and neck.

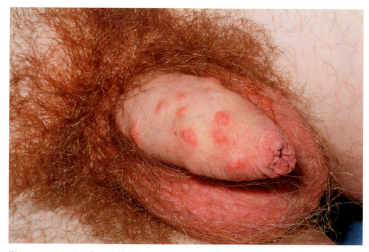

Figure 20.4: Scabietic lesions on the shaft of the penis.

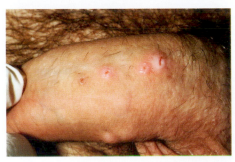

Figure 20.5: Scabietic lesions on the shaft of the penis.

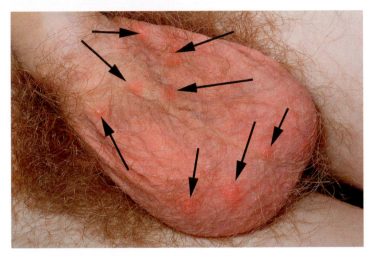

Figure 20.6: Scabietic lesions in the scrotal area.

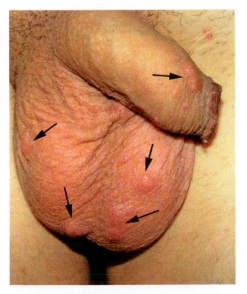

Figure 20.7: Serpiginous burrow on the shaft of the penis and nodular lesions on the scrotum.

Diagnosis

Microscopic examination of skin scraping to identify eggs or mites – larvae, nymphs or adults.

Complications

- Secondary infection.
- Acute glomerulonephritis.
- Norwegian scabies (hyperkeratotic and crusted lesions on the hands and feet).
- Nodular scabies.

Treatment

- Local
  - 5% permethrin cream local application; leave overnight and repeat after seven days. Can be used anywhere on the body except above the neck.
  - 1% gamma benzene hexachloride (Lindane) local application and repeat after seven days – contraindicated in pregnant or breastfeeding women.
  - 10% crotamiton cream (Eurax) local application, two times a day for seven days.
- Systemic
  - Ivermectin 200 mg/kg body weight, single dose.

Pruritus can be treated with antihistamines. If itching is severe, antihistamines can be prescribed. It is advisable for treatment to be administered to all family members. Routine STI screening is advisable and partners should be seen in the genito-urinary medicine (GUM) clinic.

Additional reference

Neynaber S, Wolff H. Diagnosis of scabies with dermoscopy. *CMAJ*. 2008; **178(12):** 1540–1.

Chapter 21: Pediculosis pubis

History

Pediculosis pubis is an ancient condition, which has been associated with humans for at least 10 000 years (Orion, *et al.* 2004). It was first medically documented in 1881. Pubic hair is the primary site of infestation, but other body hair may be affected.

Aetiology

Pediculosis pubis is caused by pubic lice, also called crab lice and commonly referred to as 'crabs'. They are tiny, six-legged parasitic insects approximately 2 mm to 3 mm in length, which infest pubic hair and lay eggs, called 'nits', on the hair shafts. The eggs hatch in 7 to 10 days. Pediculosis pubis may be present in other body hair, such as underarm hair, eyebrows, and rarely in eyelashes. Infestation of the eyelashes is called phthiriasis palpebrarum. Crab lice are sucking parasites which must feed on blood several times a day in order to survive.

Pubic lice belong to the species *Phthirus pubis* (Fig. 21.1), and are distinct from body lice (*Pediculus humanus corporis*) and head lice (*Pediculus humanus capitis*).

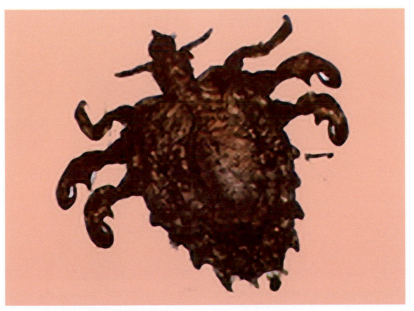

Figure 21.1: *Phthirus pubis.*

Incubation period

Following infestation, the incubation period can be between five days and several weeks, during which time the condition may be asymptomatic.

Mode of transmission

- Sexual contact.
- Close bodily contact.
- Sharing a bed with an infected person.
- Sharing clothes or towels.

Symptoms

- Nits or adult parasites may be present (Figs. 21.2 and 21.3).
- Itching of the affected area, especially at night.
- Affected area looks grey in colour.
- Skin damaged by scratching due to severe itching.

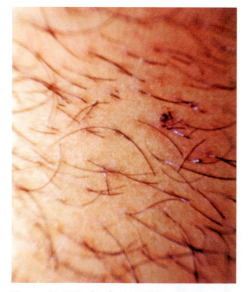

Figure 21.2: Pediculosis pubis: a louse and nits attached to the hair. (Courtesy Dr N Khanna and Mehta Publishing House)

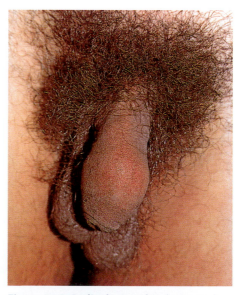

Figure 21.3: Pediculosis pubis: louse and nits attached to pubic hair. (Courtesy Dr N Khanna and Mehta Publishing House)

Diagnosis

- Clinical examination to identify nits attached to hair shafts.
- Adult parasites can be seen by magnifying glass.

Complications

Secondary infection. Pediculosis pubis may be coincident with other sexually transmitted infections.

Treatment

- Malathion 0.5% local application. Leave for 12 hours before washing out and repeat after seven days.
- Permethrin cream 5% local application. Allow to dry and wash out after 12 hours, and repeat application after seven days. It can be used for eyelashes (with the eyes closed) two times a day for 10 days.
- Phenothrin 0.5% shampoo local application; this treatment can be repeated after seven days.
- Gamma benzene hexachloride (Lindane) 1% local application and repeat after seven days.
- Ivermectin 200 mg/kg body weight administered orally once weekly for two weeks as a second line of treatment in combination with local, topical, therapy. The patient should be screened for other STIs and the partner should also be seen in the genito-urinary medicine (GUM) clinic. The importance of general hygiene should be stressed.

Additional reference

Orion E, Matz H, Wolf R. Ectoparasitic sexually transmitted diseases: scabies and pediculosis. *Clin Dermatol.* 2004; **22:** 513–9.

Chapter 22: Dermatoses affecting the genital area

22.1: Eczema

Aetiology

Eczema is a skin condition that commonly affects many parts of the body, and occasionally it may appear on the anus and female genitals. The causes may be a combination of genetic and environmental factors. If it is due to a reaction to an irritant (such as a chemical in perfumed soap), it is often referred to as dermatitis. Stress and hormonal changes may also trigger the onset of eczema.

Symptoms

Presenting symptoms are red plaques or a finely scaled skin surface. It frequently causes severe irritation and excoriation (Fig. 22.1.1). It sometimes presents as lichen simplex chronicus (Fig. 22.1.2).

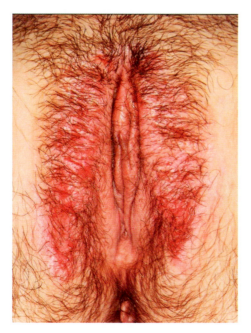

Figure 22.1.1: Eczematous lesion of vulval area.

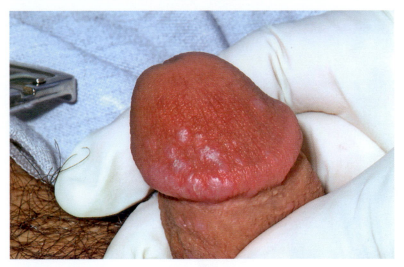

Figure 22.1.2: Lichen simplex chronicus.

Treatment

Local corticosteroid cream application is indicated.

22.2: Fixed drug eruption

Aetiology

Following oral drug therapy, fixed drug eruption causes the appearance of localised, sharply circumscribed, lesions on the skin or mucous membranes. The condition is characterised by the recurrence of the lesions at the same site each time the causative drug is administered orally. Many different drugs may induce the eruption including antibiotics (particularly sulphonamides), phenolphthalein, barbiturates, oral contraceptives and tetracycline.

Symptoms

Lesions may be erythematous, oedematous or ulcerative. They are round or oval and occasionally painful (Fig. 22.2.1, next page).

Treatment

Discontinuation of the causative drug if appropriate.

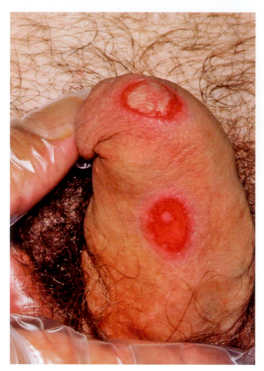

Figure 22.2.1: Fixed drug eruption.

22.3: Hair follicles and sebaceous cyst

Aetiology

Sebaceous glands are associated with hair follicles all over the body, including the shaft of the penis. They may be visible as small nodules or may look like lumps in the skin at the base of hairs. These glands secrete an oily substance called sebum. A blocked sebaceous gland can result in an accumulation of sebum and the formation of a sebaceous cyst.

Symptoms

Sebaceous cysts appear as painless lumps in the skin. If the cyst becomes infected, the lump may swell and become inflamed and tender (Fig. 22.3.1).

Treatment

Most sebaceous cysts do not require treatment, as they will resolve over time. A warm compress may help drain the cyst and speed up the healing process. Infected cysts may be treated with a steroid injection or surgically removed.

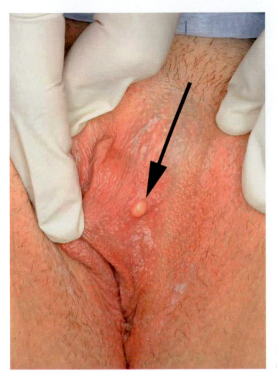

Figure 22.3.1: Sebaceous cyst in vulval area.

22.4: Lichen nitidus

Aetiology

Lichen nitidus is a rare skin condition which occasionally affects the mucous membranes and nails. The condition is characterised by skin-coloured micropapules which may resemble actinic lichen planus (that occurring on light-exposed skin). Lichen nitidus affects male and female children and young adults, but generalised variants more often affect females. In males, the micropapules are commonly present on the genitalia. The condition may co-occur with lichen planus.

Symptoms

The micropapular lesions are asymptomatic, non-itchy, flat topped and skin coloured or slightly purplish in colour (Fig. 22.4.1, next page).

Diagnosis

By clinical presentation.

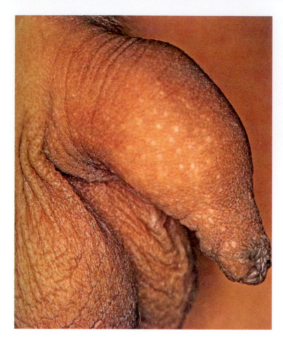

Figure 22.4.1: Lichen nitidus.

Treatment

Lichen nitidus is a self-limiting condition which recovers spontaneously and requires no treatment, although it may relapse.

22.5: Lichen planus

Aetiology

Lichen planus is a common skin condition that affects many parts of the body in males and females, including the arms, legs, mouth and genitals. People over the age of 40 years are most commonly affected, and the cause of the condition is unknown. Lichen planus is not contagious and is not transmitted during intimate contact or sexual intercourse.

Symptoms

The symptoms of this condition vary depending on the site affected.

- Skin.
  - Pruritic, violaceous, purple-coloured, flat-topped, polygonal, well-defined papular lesions (Fig. 22.5.1).

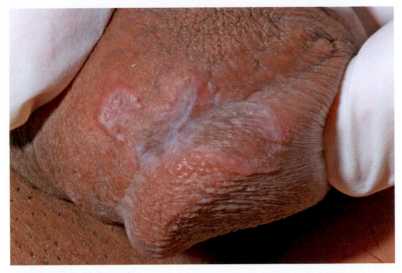

Figure 22.5.1: Lichen planus.

- – Itching – the Koebner phenomenon is common (spreading of lesions as a result of scratching).
    - – Whitish streaks (Wickham's striae) are occasionally present.
- Genitals.
    - – Angular or flat violaceous papules or plaques – on the glans, penis shaft, vulva or vagina (Fig. 22.5.1).
    - – Extreme itchiness.
    - – Yellow or greenish discharge from the vagina.
- Mouth.
    - – White and red lesions in the mouth.
    - – Pain when eating.
    - – Persistent mouth ulcers.

Diagnosis

Diagnosis can be established by clinical presentation and if necessary, biopsy for microscopic examination.

Treatment

Topical corticosteroid creams, or the topical immunomodulatory creams tacrolimus or pimecrolimus are generally effective for treatment of the skin, including the genitals. Corticosteroid sprays, mouthwashes and lozenges are available for oral lichen planus.

22.6: Genital psoriasis

Aetiology

Psoriasis is a skin condition characterised by red, scaly papules or plaques of varying sizes. Psoriasis is a chronic but non-contagious condition of unknown cause; it is thought to be an autoimmune disease.

Symptoms

Plaques are raised with sharply defined edges and silvery or whitish scales. Removal of the white scaly lesions reveals punctate bleeding spots – called Auspitz's sign (Fig. 22.6.1).

Psoriasis is most commonly present on the knees, elbows, hands, and lumbosacral region but the palms, soles, scalp, genitals, nails and joints may also be affected by the condition.

Male genitals are more frequently affected than female. Psoriasis of the genitals generally appears as well-marginated red lesions with minimal scaling, especially in circumcised males.

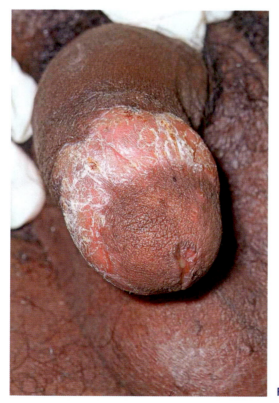

Figure 22.6.1: Psoriasis of glans penis.

Treatment

Topical corticosteroid cream is the treatment of choice. Other possible treatments include phototherapy (UVA and UVB light) and laser therapy.

22.7: Rosai–Dorfman's disease

Aetiology

Rosai–Dorfman's disease, also known as sinus histiocytosis with massive lymphadenopathy (SHML), is a rare reactive disease characterised by large, bilateral, painless lymphadenopathy, usually cervical (in the neck). The swelling of the lymph nodes is due to the accumulation of histiocytes – a type of white blood cell. In almost half of cases, at least one extranodal site is also affected which may be on the skin, bone, eyes, central nervous system or the genital area. This is a benign condition affecting young males and – less frequently – females, first described by Rosai and Dorfman in 1969.

Symptoms

Swollen lymph nodes; presenting symptoms in the urogenital area are yellow papules, plaques or nodules. Other symptoms that may be present include fever and weight loss (Fig. 22.7.1).

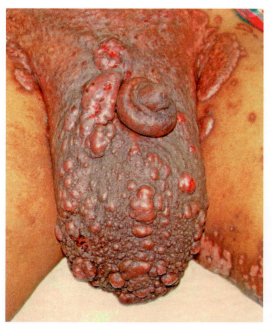

Figure 22.7.1: Rosai–Dorfman's disease.

Diagnosis

Lymph node biopsy for histological examination will confirm the diagnosis.

Treatment

Many cases resolve spontaneously, while others may require treatment such as radiotherapy, corticosteroids or cyclophosphamide (a cytotoxic agent also used to treat cancer). Despite therapy, the disease may relapse. Surgical treatment is also indicated.

22.8: Vitiligo

Aetiology

Vitiligo is a skin condition in which the pigmentation is lost in discrete patches. This is due to the loss of melanin in the skin which is normally produced by melanocytes. The aetiology is uncertain but it may be a genetic or an autoimmune disorder, possibly associated with polyglandular autoimmune syndrome which also includes a type of diabetes mellitus and thyroiditis. It may be triggered by stress, but it is not contagious and cannot be transmitted via sexual contact. The condition occurs in males and females and can affect any part of the body including the mucous membranes and the genitals, but is most common on skin exposed to light. In addition to the skin, muscles may become hypopigmented.

Symptoms

Small white patches on the skin or inside the mouth or nose; in some cases the patches become larger and merge to cover large areas of the body (Fig. 22.8.1).

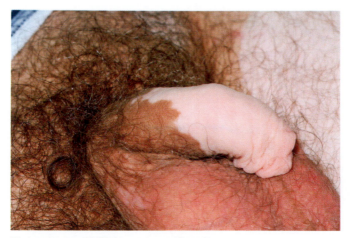

Figure 22.8.1: Vitiliginous area of penis.

Diagnosis

By clinical presentation.

Treatment

Suggested treatment includes steroid creams, although response to treatment is unpredictable and most patients do not regain the lost pigment. Treatment does not prevent the condition recurring. Cosmetics may be applied to conceal the patches.

22.9: Herpes zoster

Aetiology

Herpes zoster, also called 'shingles' is a skin rash caused by the *Varicella-zoster virus* (VZV), which is also responsible for chicken pox. After a person has recovered from chicken pox, the virus lies dormant in the nervous system where it remains indefinitely. In some people the virus becomes reactivated – often many years later – and manifests as a herpes zoster vesicular rash in a dermatomal distribution. Predisposing factors for herpes zoster include stress and immune deficiency. Anyone who has had chickenpox at any stage is at risk of developing herpes zoster. Pregnant women who have never had chicken pox may develop herpes zoster if they come into contact with someone with chicken pox or herpes zoster. This is very serious as the mother may pass the infection to the unborn child and this is potentially fatal for the foetus.

Symptoms

- Rash and burning sensation (Fig. 22.9.1, next page).
- Blisters with a red base, often itchy, along the paths of a local nerve.
- Dermatomes (areas of skin supplied by one spinal nerve) may be affected without blisters.
- Rash is usually unilateral and one nerve is involved.
- The torso is most frequently affected but the genital area may be involved, and occasionally the face.
- It may take three to four weeks for the blisters to scab and recover.
- Postherpetic neuralgia.
- Flu-like symptoms.

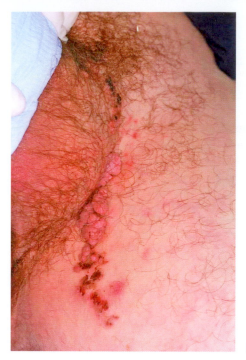

Figure 22.9.1: Herpes zoster.

Diagnosis

- Clinical picture and presentation.
- VZV can be detected in vesicular fluid by immunofluorescence method.

Treatment

Antiherpetic drugs and pain killers are effective:

- aciclovir 800 mg orally five times per day for seven days.
- valaciclovir oral therapy 1 g three times per day for seven days.
- famciclovir 300 mg orally three times per day for three days.
- NSAIDs for pain and malaise.
- amitriptyline 25 mg to 150 mg daily until symptoms subside.
- gabapentin 2.4 g daily (divided dose).

For postherpetic neuralgia:

- carbamazepine 100 mg, one or two times per day; maximum dose: 1.6 g daily.

Chapter 23: Malignant and pre-malignant conditions affecting the genital area

23.1: Erythroplasia of Queyrat (Bowen's disease of the glans penis)

History

Erythroplasia of Queyrat – also called Bowen's disease of the glans penis – is a squamous cell carcinoma of the glans penis and prepuce in uncircumcised, middle-aged, men. This condition was first described by Tarnovsky in 1891 and elaborated on by Queyrat in 1911, but only recognised as a carcinoma in 1933 by Sulzberger and Satenstein. The aetiology is unknown.

Symptoms

- One or more erythematous plaques with inflammation, crusting and scaling on the glans and prepuce (Figs. 23.1.1. and 23.1.2).

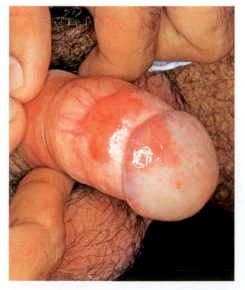

Figure 23.1.1: Erythroplasia of Queyrat: well-demarcated erythematous plaques of the glans penis and prepuce.

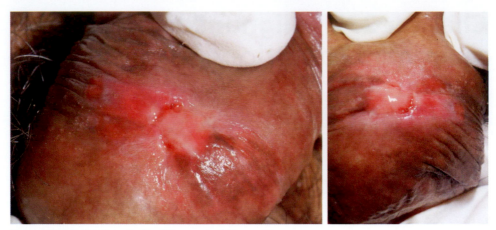

Figure 23.1.2: Erythroplasia of Queyrat of the penis.

- Ulceration.
- Pain.
- Penile discharge.
- Paraphimosis – inability to put the foreskin back over the glans (*see* also Chapter 24.7, page 147).
- Dysuria – pain when passing urine.

Single or multiple well-defined lesions that do not heal spontaneously. Ulceration may progress to squamous cell carcinoma.

Diagnosis

Diagnosis can be established by biopsy.

Treatment

Erythroplasia of Queyrat can be treated with local application of 5-fluorouracil cream (a chemotherapeutic drug). In severe or persistent cases, surgical removal of the affected tissue may be required.

23.2: Extramammary Paget's disease in the vulval area

Aetiology

Extramammary Paget's disease is a rare adenocarcinoma of the skin which is identical to Paget's disease of the breast, but occurring at a different site – including the vulva in females (it may also occur in males on the penis in extremely rare cases). The disease was first described in 1874 by Sir James Paget who detailed several cases of the condition on the female nipple, all of which had underlying breast cancer. In extramammary Paget's disease there may or may not be underlying cancer. When the disease occurs in the vulval area, there may be underlying adenocarcinoma in local glands or organs such as Bartholin's gland, the urethra or the rectum. The disease occurs most frequently in older women over the age of 60 years, and predominantly in Caucasians.

Symptoms

- Slow growing lesion – may be invasive or non-invasive, initially erythematous and dry, becoming crusted and ulcerated (Fig. 23.2.1).
- Pruritus.
- Rash.
- Pain.
- Bleeding.

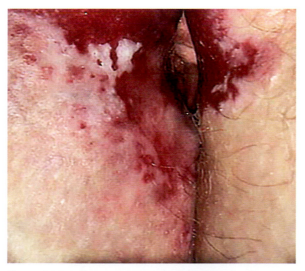

Figure 23.2.1: Extramammary Paget's disease. (Courtesy Dr John Tidy)

Diagnosis

- Clinical presentation – not alone diagnostic.
- Biopsy.

- Positive biopsy is confirmed by histological examination – presence of Paget's cells is diagnostic.

Complications

If the condition is not treated, cancer may develop.

Treatment

- Surgical removal of affected area – skin vulvectomy and split-thickness skin graft (sexual function can be preserved).
- Imiquimod 5% cream applied locally once daily for six weeks.

Treatment of complications

Extremely rare – almost all cases involving the vulva are non-invasive. If underlying cancer does occur, treatment may include:

- Surgical removal of affected tissue/organ if possible.
- Chemotherapy.
- Radiotherapy.

23.3: Squamous cell carcinoma of the glans penis

Aetiology

Squamous cell carcinoma is the most frequently occurring penile cancer. It may be present on the glans penis, prepuce or shaft of the penis and is slow growing initially, without affecting erectile function, ejaculation or urination. Consequently, many patients do not seek medical attention immediately. Several risk factors are associated with the premalignant condition, possibly predisposing the patient to squamous cell carcinoma:

- Bowen's disease of the glans penis (also called Queyrat's erythroplasia).
- bowenoid papulosis.
- human papillomavirus.
- balanitis xerotica obliterans (also called lichen sclerosus; previously lichen sclerosus et atrophicus).
- leukoplakia – a precancerous oral lesion.
- phimosis.

Staging of the disease

Staging of penile cancer was proposed by Jackson in 1966.

- Stage 1: tumour is restricted to the glans or prepuce.
- Stage 2: involvement of the penile shaft.
- Stage 3: operable metastasis of inguinal lymph node.
- Stage 4: tumour extends beyond the shaft of the penis with inoperable metastasis of inguinal lymph node.

Alternative staging of penile cancer: TNM classification, is also described in the literature.

Symptoms

Presence of a lesion that may be indurated, erythematous, nodular or ulcerous. Most cases occur in uncircumcised men so phimosis may cover the lesion. Other associated symptoms may include pain, discharge and bleeding (Figs. 23.3.1, 23.3.2 and 23.3.3).

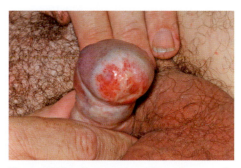

Figure 23.3.1: Squamous cell carcinoma of the glans penis.

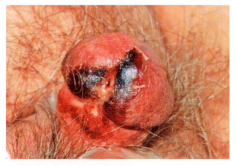

Figure 23.3.2: Squamous cell carcinoma of the glans penis.

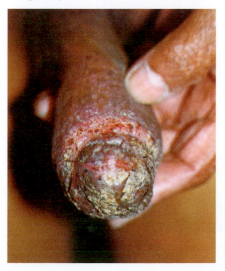

Figure 23.3.3: Squamous cell carcinoma of the glans penis. (Courtesy Dr N Khanna and Mehta Publishing House)

Diagnosis

Clinical presentation – careful examination of the lesion and palpation of lymph nodes is essential. Diagnosis is confirmed by biopsy from the lesion.

Treatment

Surgery to remove the affected tissue is essential.

23.4: Vulval carcinoma

Aetiology

Vulval carcinoma is a rare invasive malignancy – comprising only 5% of all gynaecological cancer cases – that affects the vulva of female genitalia. The carcinoma originates from the vulval epidermis – usually the labia majora – and progresses to a squamous cell carcinoma. The clitoris or fourchette may also be affected. If not addressed promptly, the squamous cell carcinoma may spread to the lymph nodes, vagina and urethra via the lymph system. The condition usually occurs in older women but may occur in younger women if risk factors are present, including smoking and human papillomavirus (HPV) infection.

Symptoms

- Lump or ulcerous lesion on the vulva (Fig. 23.4.1).
- Pruritus.

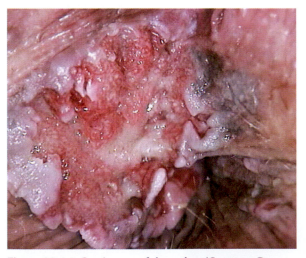

Figure 23.4.1: Carcinoma of the vulva. (Courtesy Dr John Tidy)

- Bleeding.
- Discharge.
- Dysuria – pain or discomfort when passing urine.
- Dyspareunia – pain during sexual intercourse.

Diagnosis

- Clinical presentation.
- Biopsy of the lump or lesion.
- Biopsy may be supplemented by cytoscopy and white blood cell count.

Treatment

Treatment for vulval carcinoma is based on staging of the disease:

- Stage 1: cancer is restricted to site of origin.
- Stage 2: cancer involves a small amount of neighbouring tissue or lymph nodes.
- Stage 3: cancer involves a significant amount of neighbouring tissue and lymph nodes.
- Stage 4: cancer has metastasised.

Surgical removal of affected tissue is the treatment of choice:

- Vulvectomy – removal of vulva tissue.
- Surgical removal of inguinal and femoral lymph nodes.
- Chemotherapy or radiation therapy – in advanced cases.

23.5: Pseudoepitheliomatous, keratotic and micaceous balanitis

Aetiology

Pseudoepitheliomatous, keratotic and micaceous balanitis (PEKMB) is a very rare penile skin condition first described by Lortat-Jacob and Civatte in 1966. This is a coronal balanitis which occurs in older males, usually after circumcision. PEKMB is benign or may become pseudomalignant or malignant (low grade).

Symptoms

Lesions on the glans penis are white in appearance which become crusty and keratotic; occasionally lesions resemble psoriasis. Lesions may become ulcerative, with fissuring on the glans (Fig. 23.5.1, next page).

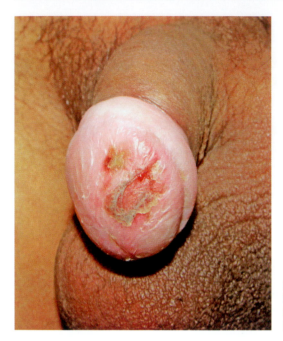

Figure 23.5.1: Pseudoepitheliomatous, keratotic and micaceous balanitis (PEKMB). (Courtesy Dr N Khanna and Mehta Publishing House)

Diagnosis

Biopsy of lesion for histological examination.

Treatment

After the biopsy result and full discussion with the patient, when there is no histological evidence of malignancy, local application of 5-Fluorouracil 5% (5-FU) cream or cryotherapy is advisable. In cases having features of atypia, extensive surgical excision such as Moh's micrographic surgery is required.

23.6: Nodular malignant melanoma of the glans penis

Aetiology

Nodular malignant melanoma of the glans penis is a rare cancer that usually affects men over the age of 50 years. Even among penile cancers, this is a rare condition. As well as the glans, the urethral meatus (opening) may be involved.

Symptoms

Black or red-brown nodules appear on the glans down to the prepuce (Fig. 23.6.1), often forming plaques and may be ulcerated. Other symptoms may include inflammation of the glans, dysuria, haematuria and discharge.

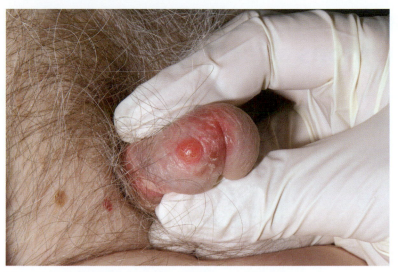

Figure 23.6.1: Nodular malignant melanoma of the glans penis.

Diagnosis

Diagnosis is often delayed in cases of nodular malignant melanoma of the glans penis due to the rarity of the disease and a frequent reluctance of patients to present their symptoms to a physician.

Diagnosis is based on the following:

- clinical presentation.
- biopsy – for histological examination.
- imaging techniques may be used to determine the extent of the disease (e.g. cytoscopy, magnetic resonance imaging – MRI).

Treatment

The choice of treatment may depend on the stage of the cancer. Penile malignant melanomas are staged as follows:

- Stage 1: cancer is restricted to the penis.
- Stage 2: cancer involves the penis and local lymph nodes.
- Stage 3: disseminated cancer – affecting other organs.

Surgical removal of affected tissue is necessary, including lymph nodes. If lymph nodes are not affected (stage 1), prophylactic removal of inguinal lymph nodes is recommended for lesions more than 1.5 mm thick. For disseminated melanoma (stage 3), chemotherapy is indicated.

Chapter 24: Miscellaneous conditions affecting the genitalia

24.1: Epidermoid cyst of the testis

Aetiology

Epidermoid cysts of the testis are uncommon benign tumours of the germ cells. The condition was first reported by Docherty and Priestly in 1942. Epidermoid cysts cannot be distinguished from malignant testicular tumours on clinical presentation and can occur at almost any age. The cyst is usually unilateral and singular.

Symptoms

Patients are usually asymptomatic except for the presence of a smooth, firm, painless testicular mass 10 mm to 30 mm in size. In some cases the patient may experience testicular discomfort and scrotal enlargement (Figs. 24.1.1 and 24.1.2).

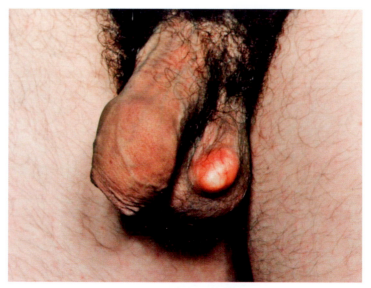

Figure 24.1.1: Epidermoid cyst in scrotal area.

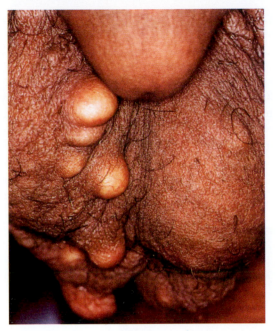

Figure 24.1.2: Multiple epidermoid cysts.

Diagnosis

The diagnosis of this condition is based on ultrasound evaluation, which should show the cyst to be within the testis parenchyma, of fibrous nature, and filled with keratinised debris.

It is necessary to exclude other masses which may occur in the scrotum, including:

- sebaceous cyst (also called an epidermal cyst) – sloughed material from the skin surface blocking a sebaceous gland, forming a cyst.
- hydrocoele – an accumulation of fluid around the testicle.
- haematocoele – a collection of blood around the testis which may be painful.
- spermatocoele (also called an epididymal cyst) – an out-pouching of tissue from the epididymis, usually containing spermatozoa.
- varicocoele – enlargement or dilation of veins in the scrotum.
- testicular tumour – a cancer common in young males and usually malignant: seminoma is the most frequently occurring type.

Treatment

Surgical treatment is always advisable for excision of the cyst, rather than complete orchidectomy.

24.2: Female circumcision

Description

Female circumcision (Fig. 24.2.1) is also called female genital mutilation (FGM) or female genital cutting (FGC). These terms refer to the practice of surgically removing females' genitalia. It is common in African countries, and also occurs in the Middle East and Asia. FMG is often performed by a traditional healer without medical training and without local anaesthesia. Consequently, the procedure is extremely painful and traumatic. The age at which FGM is carried out varies from country to country, but is usually performed on girls before puberty. The reasons for the procedure also vary and include social custom, religious requirement, and hygiene to prolong virginity or improve fertility.

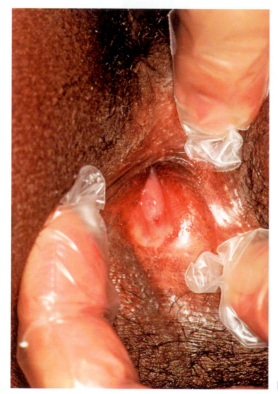

Figure 24.2.1: Female circumcision.

Procedure

During this procedure the prepuce (hood covering the clitoris), the clitoris (either partially or completely), the labia majora and labia minora are removed using a knife, scissors, razor blade or even a piece of broken glass. A small opening is left for urination and flow of menstrual fluid. Feelings of sexual arousal are either inhibited or lost completely, and sexual intercourse may be painful. Circumcised women may require caesarean section for childbirth.

Complications

There are many potential complications, some of which may be serious or even fatal, including infection, haemorrhage, sexual dysfunction and problems with pregnancy and childbirth.

24.3: Fordyce papules

Aetiology

Fordyce papules, also called Fordyce spots, is a common skin disorder that presents as tiny yellowish spots on the genitals and other sites. It is non-infectious and groups of spots may recover spontaneously. Fordyce papules are thought to be an overgrowth of sebaceous glands that are not associated with hair follicles, but the exact cause of this condition is unknown.

Symptoms

The spots are 0.5 mm to 3 mm in size. They are usually found on the penis shaft and corona, on female labia and other parts of the body, such as the lips. The spots tend to appear in groups of 50 to 100 (Fig. 24.3.1).

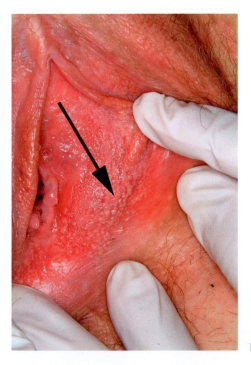

Figure 24.3.1: Fordyce's spots in female.

Treatment

These spots are harmless and no treatment is required to clear them. Tretinoin cream or gel occasionally helps for spots in cosmetic regions, and laser evaporation can be performed if required.

24.4: Hypospadias

Aetiology

Hypospadias (Fig. 24.4.1) is a congenital defect of the urethral opening in males. In this condition the urethral opening is not in its normal position at the end of the glans, but commonly opens on the ventral (underside) surface of the penis. The position of the urethral opening varies, from the base of the glans to points along the shaft and even on the perineum – behind the scrotum. The cause of this condition is not known but genetic and environmental factors may be involved.

Diagnosis

Diagnosis can be confirmed by clinical examination.

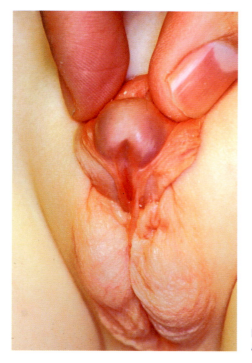

Figure 24.4.1: Hypospadias. (Courtesy of Dr Ami Lal Bhatt)

Treatment

Urinary and sexual problems are associated with this condition since the penis is often curved as a result of the deformity. Urethral stricture is sometimes present. Surgical treatment is generally successful.

24.5: Epispadias

Aetiology

Epispadias (Fig. 24.5.1) is a very rare congenital defect of the urethral meatus position that occurs in males and females, although it is more frequent in males. In males the urethra generally opens on the dorsal (upper) surface of the penis, on the side of the penis, or occasionally over the entire length of the penis rather than the tip. In females the urethral opening may be in the belly area with the urethra split along its length dorsally.

Complications

In epispadias there may be urinary tract infection and reflux – backward flow of the urine into the bladder. This may lead to reflux from the bladder to the kidneys, which may cause reflux nephropathy, resulting in kidney damage.

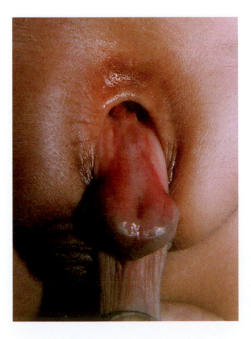

Figure 24.5.1: Epispadias. (Courtesy of Dr Ami Lal Bhatt)

Treatment

Surgical repair of epispadias is recommended.

24.6: Necrotising fasciitis

Aetiology

Necrotising fasciitis is a rare but very serious bacterial infection of the skin and soft tissue, described as fascial necrosis. It was first reported in the genitals and perineum in 1883 by Jean Alfred Fournier, after which the disease was named Fournier's gangrene, but it was given its present name of necrotising fasciitis in 1952 by Dr B Wilson. The infection usually follows tissue injury, ulceration or other minor wound.

Causative organisms

Most cases of necrotising fasciitis are multibacterial, although group A beta-haemolytic streptococci (GABS) are frequently causative, along with other streptococcal serotypes. Non-anaerobic bacteria such as *E. coli*, klebsiella and pseudomonas may also be responsible for this condition. There are three types of necrotising fasciitis, based on the types of causative organisms:

- type 1 – due to polymicrobial infection (bacteria of more than two genera).
- type 2 – due to haemolytic group A streptococci and staphylococci.
- type 3 – due to clostridial myonecrosis (*Clostridium perfringens* and *Clostridium septicum* are the causative organisms; also called gas gangrene).

Symptoms

Early symptoms occur within 24 hours.

- Erythematous lesion, swelling due to minor trauma – may be on the penis and scrotum or other sites.
- Painful ulcerative lesion (Fig. 24.6.1).
- Cellulitis.
- Flu-like symptoms.
- Formation of a black necrotic area – often in a ring around the initial lesion.
- Rapidly spreading infection along the fascial planes causing tissue death (necrosis).

The infection is very serious and should be treated as an emergency; despite treatment, many cases result in fatality.

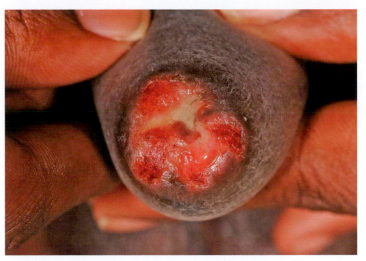

Figure 24.6.1: Necrotising fasciitis of the glans penis.

Diagnosis

- Clinical presentation.
- Biopsy of the affected tissue – to identify the causative bacterial species. Bacterial (and occasionally fungal) cultures from the infected tissue may aid diagnosis.
- Histological examination of diseased tissue – necrosis, occluded blood vessels and thrombi are diagnostic.

Treatment

- Patients should be hospitalised immediately.
- Intravenous antibiotics according to the susceptibility of bacteria – identified from gram staining of exudate.
- Surgical debridement – removal of necrotic tissue to prevent further spread of the infection.
- Intravenous immunoglobulin therapy; particularly for streptococcal infections.

24.7: Paraphimosis

Aetiology

Paraphimosis is a condition in which the prepuce (foreskin) of an uncircumcised male cannot be brought back over the head of the penis following retraction. This condition

– which is regarded as a medical emergency – occurs when the foreskin is retracted over the glans and left in that position for an extended time, during which the foreskin forms a tight constricting ring around the base of the glans. This may restrict blood flow to the glans causing oedema.

After retraction of the foreskin over the glans, the following may cause paraphimosis:

- local trauma.
- catheterisation of the penis.
- infection of the foreskin due to poor hygiene.
- allergy.

Symptoms

- Swelling (oedema) of the glans penis (Fig. 24.7.1).
- Swelling of the coronal sulcus.
- Swelling of the foreskin.
- Painful penis.
- Glans penis becomes blushed or dark coloured.

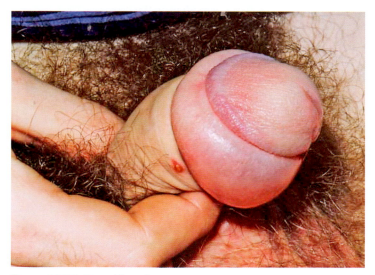

Figure 24.7.1: Paraphimosis.

Complications

Persistent paraphimosis can cause gangrene; it should be treated as an emergency by the urologist.

Treatment

The main treatment aim is to bring the foreskin back to the normal position by applying local anaesthesia – lidocaine or EMLA (lidocaine 2.5% and prilocaine 2.5%) cream – and manually pulling the foreskin back over the glans. Oral paracetamol or NSAIDs are useful to relieve pain, and sexual intercourse should be avoided for 7 to 10 days. If this treatment is unsuccessful, there is an urgent need to seek further urological advice. A dorsal slit incision or circumcision may be necessary.

24.8: Phimosis

Aetiology

Phimosis (Fig. 24.8.1) is a constriction of the male foreskin, which as a result, is unable to retract back over the glans penis. This condition may be caused by repeated infection or may be congenital – it is relatively common in male children under the age of five years.

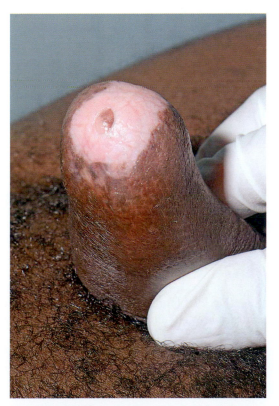

Figure 24.8.1: Phimosis associated with vitiligo.

Symptoms

Other than an inability to pull the foreskin back over the glans penis, phimosis may present as painful penile swelling, recurrent inflammation and dysuria. Phimosis is often associated with other genital conditions, most commonly balanitis – inflammation of the glans penis – due to the accumulation of sweat, urine and dead cells under the foreskin that allows bacteria to grow.

Complications

Phimosis can cause several complications including urinary problems (urinary tract infections, urinary retention), painful erection, balanitis (inflammation of the glans under the foreskin), accumulation of dead cells and bacteria under foreskin (smegma), and narrowing of the penile opening.

Treatment

Congenital phimosis usually recovers spontaneously after six months to three years. Persistent and non-congenital cases may be treated by gentle and gradual stretching of the foreskin every day for several months, and washing daily with warm water. If phimosis is troublesome and causing urinary problems, circumcision is a treatment option.

24.9: Pearly penile papules

Aetiology

Pearly penile papules are multiple tiny filiform papules that occur at the junction between the glans and the coronal sulcus of the penis. The papules or spots are acral angiofibromas. They are common in males and variants may resemble genital warts. Pearly penile papules are not contagious and cannot be transmitted during sexual contact.

Symptoms

The skin-coloured papules (Fig. 29.9.1) are 1 mm to 2 mm in size, smooth and either dome shaped or filiform, and distributed circumferentially on the corona and sulcus. The spots are otherwise asymptomatic.

Diagnosis

By clinical presentation.

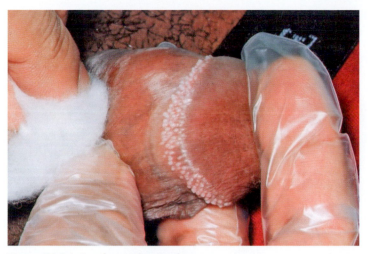

Figure 24.9.1: Pearly penile papules.

Treatment

The papules are harmless and no medical treatment is required. Patients may need reassurance that the papules are not genital warts.

24.10: Peyronie's disease

The French surgeon François Gigot de la Peyronie first described Peyronie's disease. There is scarring within the penile erectile tissue. On erection the penis bends around the scarred area resulting in a characteristic deformed appearance (Fig. 24.10.1).

Peyronie's disease is a disorder of the tunica albuginea. The scarring will often stop getting worse, but will not completely improve.

There are several treatments available like vitamin E, para-aminobenzoate, colchicine, verapamil. Direct injection of collagenase into the plaque is under investigation. High-energy radiation therapy and surgical procedures are also used. However surgery may reduce the size of the penis.

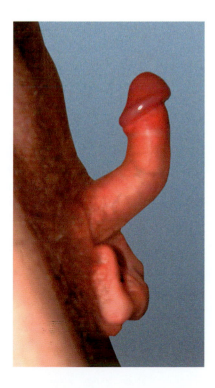

Figure 24.10.1: Peyronie's disease.

Occasionally Peyronie's disease is associated with trauma, diabetes mellitus, gout and Dupuytren's contracture. Diagnosis can be established on clinical grounds and ultrasound of the shaft of the penis, which shows hyperechoic plaques in the corpora cavernosa with acoustic shadowing suggest Peyronie's disease (Fig. 24.10.2).

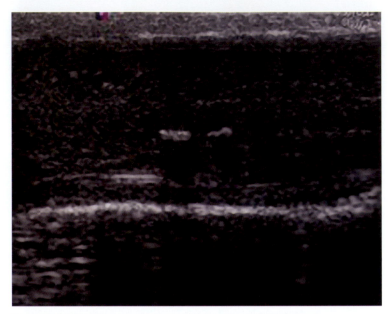

Figure 24.10.2: Ultrasound scan showing Peyronie's disease.

24.11: Artificial penile nodules

A common practice among men of eastern countries, particularly in Southeast Asia, is to use unusual materials to enhance sexual arousal and pleasure in females during intercourse. One such practice that has been documented is the implantation of artificial, non-pathological, foreign bodies under the skin of the penis shaft. These objects may be self-implanted or implanted by non-medical friends or family. They are called 'bulleetus' in the Philippines, 'chagan ball' (ball bearing) in Korea and 'tancho nodules' in Thailand.

The number of bulleetus worn by a man varies from two to six in most cases with the largest number recorded being 20. The bulleetus implants are made from a variety of materials, including plastic, polished stone, ivory, pearl or even silicone and are round or oval in shape.

Neither foreign body reactions nor secondary infections have been frequently reported. Only inflammatory reactions due to injection of silicone liquid with a syringe have been occasionally reported. These swellings might be otherwise misdiagnosed as a genital warts or sebaceous cysts (Fig. 24.11.1).

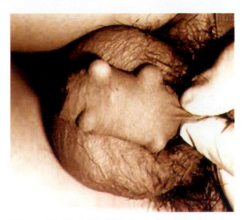

Figure 24.11.1: Artificial penile nodules (bulleetus).

24.12: Plasma cell balanitis

Aetiology

Plasma cell balanitis, also called Zoon's plasma cell balanitis or balanitis circumscripta plasmacellularis, is a rare skin condition of the penis. It was first described in 1952 by JJ Zoon and mainly affects middle-aged or older men. The aetiology of this condition is unknown but it is more common in uncircumcised males. It may be associated with friction, trauma, poor hygiene, chronic infection with *Mycobacterium smegmatis*, The same condition occurs in females, called plasma cell vulvitis or vulvitis circumscripta plasmacellularis.

Symptoms

Shiny reddish or yellow plaques appear on the glans in males and on the vulva in females. In males the condition may cause balanoposthitis – inflammation of the glans penis and prepuce (Fig. 24.12.1).

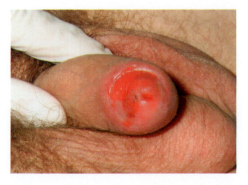

Figure 24.12.1: Plasma cell balanitis.

Diagnosis

Diagnosis is based on biopsy only – presence of plasma cell infiltrate is diagnostic.

Treatment

Topical treatments are indicated: topical antibiotic creams, antifungal creams and immunomodulatory creams (tacrolimus, pimecrolimus and imiquimod). In severe or persistent cases, urological consultation is advisable and surgical treatment (circumcision) may be advisable for males.

24.13: Priapism

Aetiology

Priapism is an unwanted painful erection that lasts for several hours – often more than four hours – without sexual arousal. The age groups usually affected are children between 5 and 10 years and adults from 20 to 50 years. JW Tripe first described the condition in 1845.

There are two types of priapism: ischaemic and non-ischaemic. In ischaemic priapism the erection is due to blood becoming trapped in the penis, because it is unable to drain back. In non-ischaemic priapism, the erection is due to an excess blood entering the penis.

There are several possible causes of priapism:

- sickle cell anaemia.
- spinal cord injury.
- a side effect of drugs to treat impotency (e.g. Viagra).
- a side effect of other drugs such as anticoagulants (e.g. warfarin, heparin), trazodone, chlorpromazine and nifedipine.
- leukaemia.
- local genital trauma.
- anaesthesia.
- pelvic tumour.

Symptoms

Painful, prolonged, erection without sexual stimulation (Fig. 24.13.1).

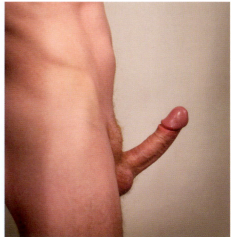

Figure 24.13.1: Priapism: painful, prolonged erection without sexual stimulation.

Diagnosis

By clinical presentation and medical history.

Complications

- Priapism may result in permanent damage and scarring to the penis within 24 hours if untreated.
- If damage occurs, an implant or prosthesis can be applied.

Treatment

The patient should be admitted to hospital immediately as it is a medical emergency requiring urgent treatment to prevent permanent damage to the penis.

- Pseudoephedrine – a decongestant drug that narrows blood vessels.
- Terbutaline – a beta agonist.
- Drain blood from the penis with a needle and syringe.
- Surgery may be needed to correct the blood flow to the penis and prevent permanent tissue damage and scarring.

24.14: Smegma

Natural history

Smegma is a thick, cheese-like, sebaceous secretion that collects under the foreskin (prepuce) in males and around the clitoris and the folds of the labia minora in females. In circumcised males it is less noticeable since smegma tends to accumulate between the base of the glans and the foreskin. Smegma is a combination of exfoliated (shed) epithelial cells and sebum, produced from sebaceous gland on the inner surface of the foreskin in males or the clitoral hood (prepuce) in females. Occasionally it has a strong odour.

Bacterial involvement

The acid-fast, gram-positive, bacterium *Mycobacterium smegmatis* has been found in smegma. This bacterium was first described in 1884 by Lustgarten, and given its present taxonomic name in 1899 by Lehmann and Neumann. *M. smegmatis* is non-pathogenic and related to other members of the *Mycobacterium* genus which cause leprosy and tuberculosis. Given that *M. smegmatis* degrades organic matter (it is also found in soil and water), it seems likely that this species survives on dead epithelial cells in smegma, rather than being responsible for producing it. The bacteria may, however, contribute to the strong odour when present.

Symptoms

Excessive accumulation of smegma (Fig. 24.14.1) in males can cause:

- balanitis – irritation and inflammation of the glans penis, causing redness and itchiness
- balanoposthitis – inflammation of the glans and the foreskin.

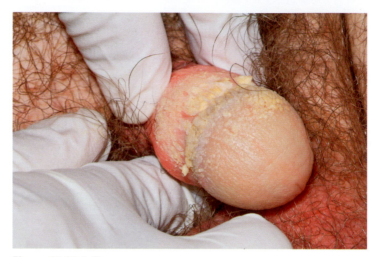

Figure 24.14.1: Smegma.

Treatment

No specific treatment is advisable except good personal hygiene, including washing daily with warm water. In cases where a male is producing unusually large amounts of smegma, circumcision should be considered.

24.15: Urethral caruncle

Aetiology

A urethral caruncle is a benign soft growth at the urethral opening in males and females. The condition is common in postmenopausal females and also occurs before puberty (when the growths are called urethral polyps), but is relatively uncommon in males.

A urethral caruncle is an outgrowth of the urethral mucosa, usually originating from the posterior lip of the urethra, and caused initially by abnormally low levels of oestrogen leading to urethral prolapse. Caruncles are covered by either squamous or transitional epithelium, and occasionally may resemble a carcinoma.

Symptoms

Urethral caruncles (Fig. 24.15.1) are usually small and asymptomatic but may reach 20 mm in size in some cases. When symptoms are present, they may be as follows:

- dysuria – difficulty or pain when passing urine.
- haematuria – blood in the urine.
- painful urethra.

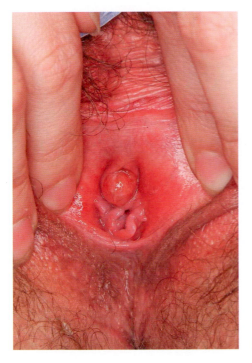

Figure 24.15.1: Urethral caruncle.

Diagnosis

By clinical presentation.

Treatment

Treatment is necessary to prevent meatal stenosis of the urethra (stricture of the urethral opening).

- Local oestrogen or anti-inflammatory cream.
- Surgical removal of the lesion.
- Catheterisation – to improve dysuria.

24.16: Urethral diverticulum

Aetiology

Urethral diverticulum is a condition that occurs in females and is a localised sac-like extension of the urethra into the tissue between the urethra and the vagina. It is usually the mid or distal part of the urethra that is affected. The urethral diverticulum is formed by enlargement of a periurethral gland. The condition was first described by William Hey in 1805 and usually occurs in women aged between 30 and 60 years old.

The cause of urethral diverticulum is not known but recurrent infection of the periurethral glands and subsequent obstruction may predispose women to the condition.

Symptoms

- Dysuria – urgent and frequent micturition (passing urine).
- Vaginal discharge.
- Dribbling when urinating.
- Dyspareunia – pain during sexual intercourse.
- Pussy discharge from the urethra.
- Blood in the urethral discharge due to infection.
- Swelling associated with urethra (Fig. 24.16.1).

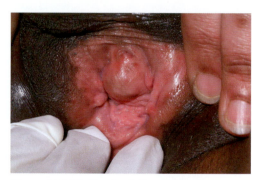

Figure 24.16.1: Urethral diverticulum.

Diagnosis

Diagnosis is based on clinical presentation and imaging techniques: ultrasound and magnetic resonance imaging (MRI).

Treatment

Surgery is the treatment of choice. Surgical options include:

- transurethral incision of the diverticular neck to widen it.
- marsupialisation by incision of the urethrovaginal septum.
- transvaginal excision to close the urethral communication with the anterior vaginal wall.

24.17: Balanitis xerotica obliterans or lichen sclerosus

Aetiology

Balanitis xerotica obliterans (BXO) (Fig. 24.17.1) – also called lichen sclerosus or LS (previously lichen sclerosus et atrophicus or LSA) (Fig. 24.17.2) – is a skin condition that primarily affects the genital area in males and females, and the anal area in females. Historically the condition was called BXO in men and LS in women. It was first described

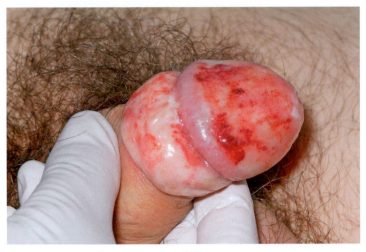

Figure 24.17.1: Balanitis xerotica obliterans.

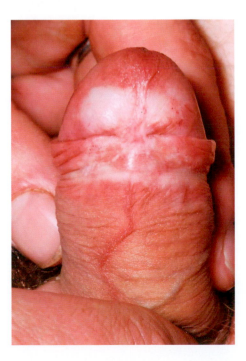

Figure 24.17.2: Lichen simplex et atrophicus.

in 1887 by François Henri Hallopeau and independently given the name balanitis xerotica obliterans in 1928 by Stuhmer, when describing the male condition. The most common age group affected is 15- to 50-year-olds, and in uncircumcised rather than circumcised males.

BXO/LS is a chronic inflammatory skin disease of unknown cause, but genetic factors and autoimmune processes may be involved. In men, the foreskin and glans penis are mainly affected, whereas in females the vulva and anal areas are affected, although other parts of the body are occasionally affected.

Symptoms

- Males (BXO)
  - Lesions on the glans and prepuce (Figs. 24.17.2, previous page, and 24.17.3) – these are discrete, angular, white, atrophic macular patches.
  - Pruritus.
  - Tenderness.
  - Painful erection.
  - Painful micturition (passing urine).
  - White papules in non-genital areas.
- Females (LS)
  - Lesions on the vulva (Figs. 24.17.4 and 24.17.5) and anus – these are white, raised, papules, plaques or atrophic patches.
  - Itching – the Koebner phenomenon is common (spreading of lesions as a result of scratching).
  - Painful micturition (passing urine).
  - Painful defaecation.
  - Thinning of the skin in the anogenital area.

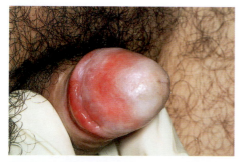 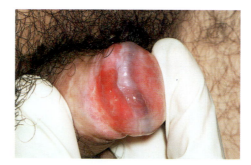

Figure 24.17.3: Lichen simplex et atrophicus.

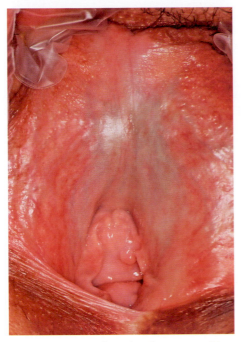

Figure 24.17.4: Lichen simplex et atrophicus.

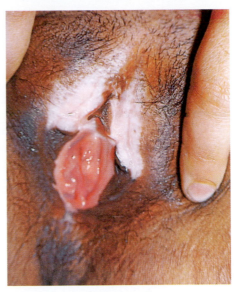

Figure 24.17.5: Lichen simplex et atrophicus with vulval lesions and narrowing of introitus. (Courtesy Dr N Khanna and Mehta Publishing House)

- Loss of skin pigmentation.
- White papules in non-genital areas.

Diagnosis

Diagnosis can be established by aetiology and clinical presentation.

Complications

If left untreated, BXO in males can cause phimosis or paraphimosis, and it may be a contributing factor for the development of penile cancer.

Treatment

In males BXO can be treated with antibiotics, corticosteroid cream, or laser therapy. In severe cases, circumcision is the most effective treatment. In females, local application of corticosteroid cream, tacrolimus and pimecrolimus creams (topical immunosuppressants) are indicated.

24.18: Vaginismus

Aetiology

Vaginismus is an involuntary tightening of the vagina during attempted intercourse, which makes it difficult to perform normal penetration. It is caused by spasm of the pelvic muscles and contraction of the muscles around the lower part of the vagina. The tightening of the muscles may be so extreme that the vagina closes completely and penetration is impossible. The cause of the condition may be psychological (due to abuse, or to an early bad experience with attempted sex or vaginal examination) or the result of an infection or injury to the vagina or bladder.

Symptoms

There are two types of vaginismus:

1 Primary – sexual intercourse has never been possible due to tightening of the vagina, pain when attempting sex, impossible to achieve penetration, discomfort and ongoing pains due to unknown origin.

2 Secondary – difficulty achieving penetration in women who have previously had a history of sexual intercourse. This can occur at any age but usually occurs later in life; it is characterised by vaginal tightness and painful penetration.

This condition makes it difficult to examine the patient with a speculum, especially for a cervical smear.

Diagnosis

Using detailed history and symptoms. A physical examination may not be possible.

Treatment

- Vaginal dilators – these can progressively stretch the muscles around the vagina.
- Psychosexual counselling – to address any underlying psychological causes.
- Relaxation therapy.

24.19: Vestibulitis

Aetiology

Vestibulitis (also referred to as vestibulodynia) was first described in 1988 by Edward Friedrich, and has symptoms similar to vulvodynia and vaginismus. With vestibulitis a patient experiences pain and discomfort in the vestibular area – the part of the vulva between the labia minora. This area contains the vaginal and urethral openings, Bartholin's glands (which produce a lubricating secretion), and small mucus-secreting vestibule glands. The condition is often chronic and may persist for several years.

Causes

The cause of vestibulitis is usually unknown, but some cases may be due to sensitivity to soaps, other bath products or treatment for an infection, or may follow childbirth. The human papillomavirus may also be implicated in some cases.

Symptoms

- Pain in the vaginal area – may occur with sexual intercourse, when inserting a tampon, or just when touched gently.
- Burning sensation and irritation of the vestibule.
- Frequent micturition (passing urine).

Diagnosis

Diagnosis is based on history, as there may be no visible symptoms.

Treatment

- Vitamin A and D ointment – local application to ease discomfort.
- Lidocaine 5% gel or cream – local application for pain relief; can be applied before sexual intercourse.
- EMLA cream (lidocaine and prilocaine) – local topical anaesthetic.
- Calcium nitrate 1200–1800 mg orally once daily – may help prevent the condition.

24.20: Vulvodynia

Aetiology

Vulvodynia is vulvar pain without any known specific cause. The condition has symptoms similar to those of vestibulitis and vaginismus; in all of these conditions discomfort and pain are the main complaints. In vulvodynia the pain may occasionally extend to the vestibule region, in which case it may be described as vulvar vestibulitis syndrome. The pain may be acute initially, but often becomes chronic and may persist for several years. It can affect women of almost any age and is not associated with abnormal gynaecology.

Causes

The cause of vulvodynia is usually unknown, but it is not associated with sexually transmitted infection (STI). However, it is not clear whether candida or trauma, (possibly to the spine) are involved.

Symptoms

Common complaints may be as follows:

- sudden onset of vulval pain.
- tenderness in the labial area (Fig. 24.20.1).
- burning, itching and discomfort in vulval area.
- dyspareunia – pain during or after sexual intercourse.
- difficulty inserting tampons.

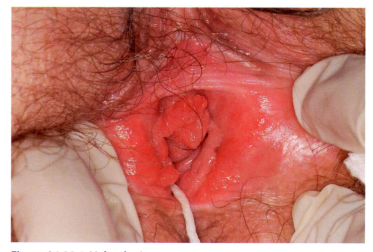

Figure 24.20.1: Vulvodynia.

Diagnosis

Based on history as there may be no visible symptoms.

Treatment

- Lubricant application – to ease discomfort during intercourse.
- Topical steroid ointment – 2.5% hydrocortisone ointment or 0.1% triamcinolone ointment to ease irritation and pain.

- Amitriptyline (tricyclic antidepressant) therapy – up to a maximum of 75 mg orally, once daily.
- Alternatives: paroxetine or venlafaxine for patients intolerant to amitriptyline.
- Nortriptyline – as for amitriptyline.
- Gabapentin – up to 1200 mg (300 mg four times per day) for pain relief.
- Lidocaine 5% gel or cream – before sexual intercourse for local pain relief.

24.21: Cervical polyp

Aetiology

Cervical polyps are small soft growths that protrude from the mouth of the cervix in the neck of the womb (Fig. 24.21.1).

Symptoms

- Bleeding after intercourse.
- Bleeding between periods.
- Abnormally heavy bleeding during menstrual cycle.
- Bleeding after menopause.

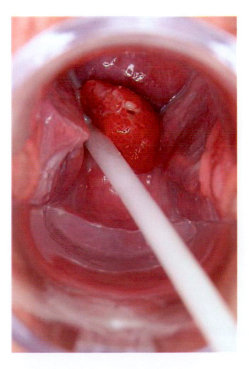

Figure 24.21.1: Cervical polyp.

Treatment

Polyps can be removed during surgical procedure or by electrocautery. Sometimes polyps can be confused with cervical warts.

24.22: Behçet's disease

Aetiology

Behçet's disease is a syndrome resulting from inflammation of the blood vessels (vasculitis), primarily in three areas: the mouth, genitals, and eyes (uveal tract specifically), although other parts of the body may be affected including the skin, joints and nervous system. The disease causes ulceration of the mouth and the genitals, uveitis, and lesions or inflammation at the other affected sites. Behçet's disease was first described in 1937 by the Turkish dermatologist, Hulusi Behçet. The aetiology is unknown but it may be an autoimmune disease, possibly triggered by infection.

Symptoms

It is very uncommon for patients to present with the full range of symptoms. Potential symptoms are:

- oral aphthous ulcers – may be on the tongue, lips (Figs. 24.22.1), gums or inside the cheeks.
- genital sores – may occur anywhere in the groin area but in males these usually appear on the scrotum and glans penis (Fig. 24.22.2); in females they occur on the cervix, vulva or vagina.

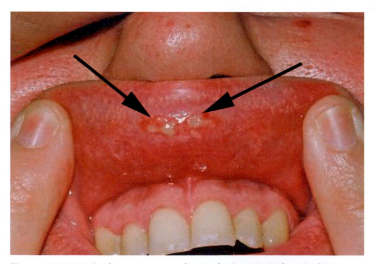

Figure 24.22.1: Oral mucous membrane lesions in Behçet's disease.

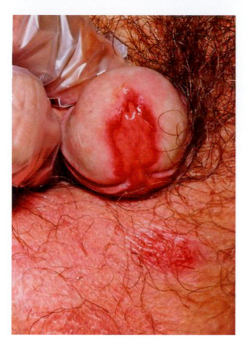

Figure 24.22.2: Penile ulceration in Behçet's disease.

- skin lesions (erythema nodosum) – usually on the face or lower limbs.
- eye inflammation – anterior uveitis (inflammation of the iris, ciliary body and choroid).
- swelling of the joints – typically the wrists, ankles and knees.
- central nervous system inflammation – this causes headache, muscle tremor, incontinence, double vision and unilateral paralysis.
- gastrointestinal inflammation – this causes vomiting, diarrhoea and abdominal pain.

Diagnosis

- Clinical presentation – at least three episodes of mouth ulcers within 12 months, in addition to other symptoms.
- HLA-B51 is associated with Behçet's disease, although this is not routinely tested.

Complications

If untreated Behçet's disease may lead to severe complications of the eye and the brain.

Treatment

- Colchicine – administered orally for mouth and genital ulcers.
- NSAIDs – to relieve pain and reduce inflammation.
- Steroid drops for eyes – to reduce uveitis.
- Oral steroids – to reduce inflammation.
- Cyclosporine – oral immunosuppressant.
- Azathioprine – oral immunosuppressant.
- Chlorambucil – oral immunosuppressant, used in combination with corticosteroids.

24.23: Vulvitis

Aetiology

Vulvitis is inflammation of the vulva in females, due to infection, irritation, allergic reaction or physical trauma. The area affected may include the labia (majora and minora), clitoris and urethral and vaginal openings. If the vaginal opening is involved, the condition may also be referred to as vulvovaginitis.

The most common causes of vulvitis are irritation or allergic reaction to soaps and sprays used on the vulval area, or to detergents used to wash underwear and sanitary towels. Other common causes are fungal infections such as *Candida albicans* (*see* Chapter 12, page 63), bacterial infections such as gardnerella (*E. coli*, mycoplasma and staphylococci may also be causative) and viral infections such as genital herpes (*see* Chapter 16, page 84). Infestations such as scabies (*see* Chapter 20, page 112) and pediculosis (*see* Chapter 21, page 117) may also cause vulvitis.

Risk factors include wearing tight synthetic underwear, poor personal hygiene, riding horses or bicycles, diabetes and being postmenopausal (loss of oestrogen leads to drying and thinning of the vulval tissue).

Symptoms

Any or all of the following symptoms may be present:

- pruritus of the vulva.
- burning sensation.
- redness and swelling.
- fissures in the skin.
- fluid-filled blisters.
- redness and swelling in vulval area (Fig. 24.23.1).

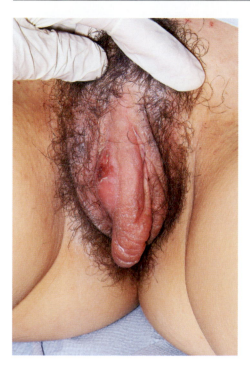

Figure 24.23.1: Vulvitis: redness and swelling in vulval area.

- skin thickening and whitening.
- vaginal discharge.

Diagnosis

- Clinical presentation.
- Vaginal swab if discharge is present, for microscopic examination – this will identify a bacterial or fungal infection.
- Culture of vaginal discharge to identify causative bacterial, fungal or viral infection.
- Lesion biopsy – may identify infestations or allergy.
- Pap smear – may identify low oestrogen levels.

Complications

Vulvitis may be a symptom of a sexually transmitted infection or a precancerous condition of the vulva. If these are suspected, the patient should be screened and biopsied as appropriate and treated accordingly.

Treatment

If the cause is an allergy to soap or detergent used for washing underclothes then no treatment is required other than avoidance of the products in question. If the cause is an infection or hormone imbalance, the following treatments are indicated:

- corticosteroid cream – local application for pruritus.
- antibiotics – for bacterial infections; the choice of antibiotic depends on the causative species.
- antifungal creams – applied locally for candida and other fungal infections; usually one of the following: clotrimazole, nystatin or miconazole.
- oral antihistamines – for cases caused by severe allergic reaction.
- oestrogen replacement therapy – for postmenopausal vulvitis.
- premarin 0.625 mg/g vaginal cream – local application for postmenopausal vulvitis.

Appendix

SHHAPT: Sexual Health and HIV Activity Property Type
Definitions and codes used in the United Kingdom's National Health Service

SHHAPT (KC60) Code Look-Up
Summary of definitions

A. DIAGNOSIS OF INFECTION, CONDITION OR DISEASE

DIAGNOSIS		SHHAPT CODE	DIAGNOSIS		SHHAPT CODE
Chlamydia		C4	Hepatitis A	Acute infection	C15
Gonorrhoea		B	Hepatitis B	First diagnosis	C13
Syphilis	Primary	A1	Hepatitis C	First diagnosis	C14
	Secondary	A2	Chancroid		C1
	Early latent	A3	LGV		C2
	Cardiovascular	A4	Donovanosis		C3
	Neurosyphilis	A5	Trichomoniasis		C6A
	Other late and latent	A6	Scabies		C8
	Congenital	A7A	Pediculosis pubis		C9
Non specific genital infection		C4N	Molluscum contagiosum		C12
Genital herpes	First episode	C10A	PID and epididymitis		C5A
	Recurrent episode	C10B	Ophthalmia neonatorum		C5B
Genital warts	First episode	C11A	BV and anaerobic balanitis		C6B
	Recurrent episode	C11D	Balanitis/vaginitis/vaginosis	Other causes	C6C
HIV	Known positive	H	Candidosis		C7
	New diagnosis	H1	Urinary tract infection		D2A
	New diagnosis – acute infection	H1A	Other conditions requiring treatment		D2B
	New diagnosis – late infection	H1B	Cervical cytology	Minor	P4A
	Attendance for HIV related care	H2		Major	P4B

B. SERVICES PROVIDED

SERVICE PROVIDED		SHHAPT CODE	SERVICE PROVIDED		SHHAPT CODE
STI tests	Chlamydia only	T1	Cervical cytology done		P4
	Chlamydia and gonorrhoea	T2	Partner notification	Initiated*	PN
	Chlamydia, gonorrhoea and syphilis	T3		Chlamydia	PNC
	Chlamydia, gonorrhoea, syphilis & HIV	T4		Gonorrhoea	PNG
HIV test	Antibody test	P1A		Syphilis	PNS
	Test offered and refused	P1B		HIV	PNH
	Test not appropriate	P1C	PEPSE		PEPS
Hepatitis B vaccination	1st dose	P2A	Contraception		P3
	2nd dose	P2B	No service and/or no treatment required		D3
	3rd dose	P2C	Prisoner		Z
Hepatitis B immune		P2I	Sex worker		SW
HPV vaccination	1st dose	W1			
	2nd dose	W2			
	3rd dose	W3			

C. SUFFIXES TO SHHAPT CODES

DESCRIPTION	WITH SHHAPT CODE	SUFFIX	DESCRIPTION	WITH SHHAPT CODE	SUFFIX
Rectal infection	B, C4, C2, C4N	R	Medication given*	B, C4, C10A, C10B, C11A, C11D	M
Pharyngeal infection	B, C4, C2	O	Quadrivalent HPV vaccine	W1, W2, W3	Q
Patient diagnosed previously elsewhere	B, C4, H1, H1A, H1B	X			

*For use in Level 2 and level 1 services only.

Index